The PSILOCYBIN HANDBOOK for Women

How Magic Mushrooms, Psychedelic Therapy, and Microdosing Can Benefit Your Mental, Physical, and Spiritual Health

JENNIFER CHESAK

Published by:
ULYSSES PRESS
PO Box 3440
Berkeley, CA 94703
www.ulyssespress.com

ISBN: 978-1-64604-498-6
Library of Congress Control Number: 2023930760

Printed in the United States
10 9 8 7 6 5 4 3 2

Acquisitions editor: Kierra Sondereker
Project editor: Renee Rutledge
Managing editor: Claire Chun
Editor: Scott Calamar
Front cover design: Rebecca Lown
Interior design: what!design @ whatweb.com
Artwork: © EnkaArts/shutterstock.com
Layout: Winnie Liu

For Mom and Dad

CONTENTS

WHY a BOOK for Women?

You are the medicine.

—María Sabina Magdalena García

Fun fact: women report more frequent use of some psychedelics than men.

A not-so-fun fact: in the Global Drug Survey 2020,[1] women cite depression, anxiety, relationship issues, trauma, and post-traumatic stress disorder (PTSD) as their main reasons for using psychedelics. Additional reasons include other mental health disorders, grief, distress over medical conditions, and chronic-pain. The truth is that more women report self-treating with some psychedelics than men.

None of this surprises me.

People assigned female at birth are two to three times more likely to develop PTSD than those assigned male at birth.[2] And most chronic-pain conditions are more prevalent in people assigned female at birth.[3] Yet healthcare providers, and people in general, are more likely to take women's pain less seriously than the pain of men.[4] For decades, medical science has either underrepresented women or left us out entirely in studies.[5] Women were even excluded from early-stage clinical trials—for the most part—until the 1990s.[6] Yes, the 1990s, people! Research on conditions that either disproportionately affect those assigned female at birth or that solely affect them is also woefully underfunded.[7] Plus, research on women's health often takes what's been referred to as a "bikini approach."[8] When research does focus on us, it tends to home in on reproductive health, ignoring other aspects.[9]

I've had firsthand experience with a chronic-pain condition that desperately needs more research. This condition impacts 10 percent of people of reproductive age who were assigned female at birth,[10] does not have a cure—or adequate treatments—and takes 10 years on average to receive a diagnosis.[11]

In the early aughts, I was diagnosed with endometriosis. I also have chronic migraine. Nothing—aside from a hysterectomy in 2016—has brought me more enduring relief for both conditions than edibles. Specifically, I ingest small quantities of delta-9-tetrahydrocannabinol (THC), the most well-known psychoactive cannabinoid in cannabis, often called marijuana (when the plant has high enough concentrations of THC). It took me nearly 20 years to not only figure out that THC helped me but to also glean regular access to it.

Lest you think I don't know my plant-based substances, not everyone considers cannabis to be a classic psychedelic—but many do, and it can have some psychedelic effects,[12] especially at high doses. Regardless of what drug camp you put marijuana in, the cannabis landscape offers us a look at how drugs that were once considered to be mainly recreational (not to mention illegal) can eventually be considered therapeutic *and* legal—at least in some places. If you've been paying attention to the landscape of psychedelics, you're likely aware that they're undergoing a research renaissance right now, especially as potential therapy (with some caveats) for mental health issues, substance use disorders, trauma, and even chronic-pain.[13]

In writing this book, I'm not suggesting that everyone who has a physical or mental health condition run out and start using psilocybin, better known as "magic mushrooms." That would be irresponsible of me.

And I'm not that kind of girl.

I *am* the type of girl who does her research—like a lot of it. I'm a medical journalist and fact-checker, and I've researched psilocybin at length, specifically how psilocybin affects and may help women or people assigned female at birth, whether therapeutically, spiritually, or recreationally. You'll find a synthesis of that research—along with personal stories, including my own—in these pages.

A shroom of one's own

That subheading is courtesy of a friend who has been entertaining me with alternative titles for this book. When I've told people I'm writing a book about psilocybin, some have asked, "Why is it for women?"

Preliminary research suggests that magic mushrooms may affect people assigned female at birth differently than those assigned male at birth.[14] Plus, a host of health conditions impact people assigned female at birth disproportionately, differently, or solely. And we deserve a book that addresses what role, if any, psilocybin therapy may be able to play.

I'm not the type of girl to exclude anyone. While this book has content specific to those assigned female at birth, it's also a resource for everyone. Often the language reporting data in medical studies is binary, using terms like *men*, *women*, *male*, and *female*. I can't change the way medical studies report on data. However, I recognize that gender isn't a binary construct. I'm opting to use inclusive language as much as possible. For example, you'll see *breastfeeding* and *chestfeeding* used together. You'll also see places where I'm leaning into my personal feminine identity as I write this book. These language strategies are an imperfect solution. Just as we need more research for conditions that affect people assigned female at birth, we also need more data specific to people who are nonbinary.

My intent is to guide you through the growing body of research regarding psilocybin's potential and provide you the safety details and considerations should you choose to use magic mushrooms.

I'm doing all of this in a decidedly bro-free format. No mushroom mansplaining here. That may sound snarky. And it is. The mushroom is the true teacher here, anyway. However, the psychedelics space *does* have a history of excluding women, discounting their scientific and other contributions, and silencing their voices.[15] So I've opted to elevate the voices and work of female and nonbinary clinicians, scientists, healers, and psychonauts in this book. Plus, mansplaining is a thing. And it's an annoying thing at that. Case in point: When I first told a much-beloved guy friend over text I was writing about psilocybin, he was thrilled. But he also took a moment to inform me that the mushroom emoji I had sent in celebration was not, in fact, psilocybin. (Bruh, I love you, but it was the only mushroom emoji on my phone!)

In this book, I've also included content about sexual health and psilocybin. (You'll find that in Chapter Six.) This topic is of particular importance, since women are disproportionately affected by sexual dysfunction.[16] Anecdotal evidence shows that psychedelics may have sex-life enhancing effects.[17] Any convo about sex and drugs, however, also requires robust content about consent, especially when we consider that the psychedelics industry has an abuse-of-power problem.[18]

Us gals are busy AF.

In between deadlines and tasks, I've at times asked myself, *Do I have time to pee?* That's why I've written this book in such a way as to provide you the information you want for your situation right now, whether you're a psychedelic newbie or seasoned psilonaut. In Chapter Two, for example, you'll find frequently asked questions coupled with quick-hit answers, plus recommendations for further reading within the book. At any time, you can also peruse the "choose your own adventure"–style table of contents to access the info you need. Chapter Eight is all about parenting and psilocybin, for example. Once at your chapter destination, you'll be able to choose your next info adventure by following the prompts—whether you need a microdose of content or a full-on topical deep dive.

As women, we're busy because we perform some of the most crucial roles in society. When compared to men, women do disproportionately more of the unpaid work of general life.[19] Yep, that's not true in every situation. Many men out there do their fair share of unpaid domestic and emotional labor, as well. But, hey, I'm trying to draw a cool parallel between women and fungi. So just go with it (and don't increase my emotional labor by sending me hate DMs, please). Women tend to be some of society's biggest doers, nurturers, and connectors. And fungi perform these same roles for nature, specifically for plant and soil ecosystems.

An estimated 5.1 million species of fungi exist, and many are crucial for the survival of up to 80 percent of plant species.[20] Fungi grow filaments of hyphae that form mycelium, ultimately connecting plants to each other in the soil. A whole forest, for example, is connected by a mycorrhizal network, or what's been dubbed the "wood wide web." Writing her doctoral thesis at the time, Suzanne Simard, PhD, now a professor of forest psychology, discovered the network in 1997.[21] Go, Dr. Simard! Why the wood wide web? Fungi exchange nutrients with soil and plants and even transfer nutrients from plant to plant, sending resources where they're needed most. If one area of the forest has struggling trees, for example, those trees can get a nutrient infusion from another section, all via this natural nexus—thanks to fungi, which also benefit from the community and collaboration.[22] When I think about magic mushrooms and the way they can sometimes make us feel more connected to each other and nature at large, my mind is officially blown.

Just to recap though: Women are super busy doing unpaid labor in addition to all their paid labor. Meanwhile, they're disproportionately affected by chronic-pain conditions and certain types of trauma. Yet society and the medical establishment have a history of ignoring women's health. Wow. Maybe fungi—nature's nurturers—can help us gals out.

Notes on legal status, stigma, and hopes for the future

In the mid-'90s, as a teen, I was driving my hot, hot Chevy Celebrity when one of my passengers yelled, "We gotta go back!" His dose of lysergic acid diethylamide (LSD)—or it might have been the whole blotter paper (the details are hazy)—had gone out the window. (In case you are wondering, we did not find his acid. But he had more.) This experience was my first encounter with psychedelics. But I did not partake. I didn't partake when some of my friends drank mushroom tea, and I didn't partake when they smoked weed either.

I was kind of the mother hen of the group, keeping a watchful eye over everyone else. (I was a trip sitter before I knew the term.) Plus, I lived in rural North Dakota and always had to drive a good distance to get home. Remaining sober just seemed like the best plan for me and certainly anyone else on the road. I also wasn't comfortable being in such an altered state of mind. What if I had a bad experience? Back then, I didn't have the information to help me navigate any potential hurdles I might encounter while getting high or tripping. A book like this wasn't available to me at my local library. And internet research in 1995 wasn't quite what it is today.

Back in the '90s, cannabis and psychedelics were highly illegal all over the United States. In the previous decade, the Reagan administration had expanded the Nixon administration's war on drugs,[23] fueling a hysteria about rampant substance abuse, which didn't really exist. The situation was akin to the satanic panic,[24] the conspiracy theory in the 1980s that devil worshipping was also pervasive. (Dang, people were paranoid in the latter part of the twentieth century, eh?) The pandemonium about out-of-control drug use further fueled stigma about illicit substances, including cannabis and psychedelics. I bring this up because the government's vilifying and mainstream society's stigmatization of these substances (and others) have done a disservice to people. I'd be remiss not to mention the devastating consequences incarceration for drug offenses—for substances that now have scientific evidence of being therapeutic—have had (and are still having) on people of color.[25] I'd also be remiss not to mention that 80 percent of the legalized cannabis market, which is projected to top $100 billion globally by the next decade,[26] is controlled by white business owners.[27] We're seeing a similar whitewashing occur with psychedelics: it's a concern regarding medical studies,[28] and it's a concern in the marketplace.[29]

The war on drugs also caused research on both cannabis and psychedelics to stall out for years, delaying some of the exciting things scientists are in the process of studying and have recently uncovered. For example, now that psychedelics are being studied for substance use disorder,[30] I can't help but wonder if widely available psilocybin therapy for addiction could have staunched some of the opioid epidemic that so many of us, including myself, have lost loved ones to. I have more what-ifs. But we can't go back and undo the harm that's been done. We can only go forward and replace disinformation with facts. We can work to eradicate stigma and advocate for decriminalization. (More on this in Chapters Eight and Ten.)

I don't regret my decision to abstain from cannabis and psychedelics back then, because ultimately, I *did* have a bad experience in the mid-aughts. I was suffering from chronic-pain from endometriosis. (Dear reader, if you deal with this, I'm sorry.) I had a prescription for opioids from a pain clinic at the time. But the pills made me too queasy and fuzzy to concentrate at work, so I generally took the medication only in the most desperate of situations. Looking back now, I'm thankful for my weak stomach. I easily could have become another victim of the opioid epidemic, which was really ramping up at the time.[31] (Prescription opioids do have an important role in pain management, but the way my pain doctor doled them out was questionable.)

I needed a more viable and regular solution. A friend suggested I try marijuana. I have severe asthma, however, and had never smoked anything in my life. (I know—what a square!) When I took a hit from a bowl (a small pipe), it burned my lungs and caused a bronchospasm, also known as an asthma attack. I grabbed my albuterol inhaler, took a puff, and held it in. What happened next was terrifying. For anyone not overly familiar with cannabis, please keep in mind that THC (the legit stuff, not the synthetic kind) is one of the least toxic of recreational drugs.[32] I just wanted to provide that note so as not to spread irrational fears. The albuterol dilated my airways and likely gave me a bigger hit than I bargained for. I experienced brief myoclonic (involuntary) jerking and longer-lasting intense anxiety. The experience, although ultimately benign, was something I never wanted to repeat.

Why am I sharing the story of what amounted to a pot freak-out in what's supposed to be a book about magical fungi? Again, the trajectory of the cannabis landscape gives us a glimpse at what the future might hold for psychedelics. I didn't try THC again for another decade, with much better success in edible form. What I've found is that I like to microdose. Microdosing is exactly what it sounds like, taking a small dose, usually regularly or semi-regularly. Microdosing THC helps me sleep better (I've always had insomnia), seems to help prevent my migraine attacks and lessen their severity, and provides me with relief from endometriosis pain. (These are simply my personal experiences; they may be different for you.)

Perfectly portioned THC gummies are obviously now available at dispensaries in US states (and elsewhere globally) that have legalized marijuana for medicinal purposes, recreational purposes, or both. I can even seek out and access, for most products, the certificate of analysis from an independent lab and see what's in it, including the percentage of each major cannabinoid, such as THC. I can take the exact amount of THC I want and dose up from there if I'm looking for an additional effect. Plus, I don't have to smoke or make my own weed brownies, trying to figure out portions. And I don't have to have a dealer—except my husband who goes to the dispensary for me when I'm too busy. Did I mention women are busy?

I know what you're thinking: *Enough with the weed talk, lady! I came here to read about shrooms.*

I'm hoping we get to a similar level with psychedelics—where they, too, can feel like less of an unknown to people. It took me decades of suffering with endometriosis and chronic migraine, tens of thousands of dollars in medical bills, countless missed days of work, and countless missed times out with friends or family to finally arrive at a solution that brings me relief. I'm not saying all my issues would have been alleviated if I'd had better access to THC earlier. But I do think my chronic-pain trajectory would have been different. The legal status, the stigma, and more were all barriers to THC for me. I was also concerned my doctors wouldn't prescribe needed medications if they detected marijuana in my system on urinalysis, whether at the clinic or the emergency room (where I landed often). This fear was not unwarranted, considering the Centers for Disease Control and Prevention (CDC) only changed guideline recommendations on testing patients for marijuana in 2016.[33] But this all relates to stigma.

Many people out there are likely grappling with similar concerns about magic mushrooms. I don't mean regarding testing. (See Chapter Two for info about that.) But the point remains. Magic mushrooms aren't decriminalized or legalized everywhere, and stigma is still a barrier. Legal concerns and stigma likely prevent people who could potentially benefit from psilocybin from accessing or using it.

Psilocybin is in the middle of a research renaissance right now. Scientific evidence on therapeutic use is expanding all the time, but it still has a long way to go. I don't want to erroneously position psilocybin as a miracle cure for every ailment under the sun. *That* it is not. Neither is cannabis. I also don't want to over-Westernize or overmedicalize what's considered a sacred substance.

Indigenous people have used psilocybin in ceremonies, rituals, and celebrations for thousands of years. As scientific research moves forward, we don't want to leave out Indigenous wisdom, which also provides valuable insight. (See Chapter Eleven.) Plus, Indigenous wisdom introduced us to psilocybin in the first place. (You can read about that introduction in Chapter Twelve, though it's not a pretty story, because it's about colonialism.) We also don't want to discount the mystical aspect of magic mushrooms. They are pretty magical!

I'm here to provide you with the latest research. And I'm incorporating knowledge from the experts studying and administering psilocybin in clinical trials, mental health professionals with expertise in psilocybin-assisted therapy, researchers who focus on harm reduction, healers employing Indigenous wisdom, women who are currently using or have used shrooms for all sorts of reasons, and more.

I hope the information in these pages empowers you to make the best decisions for yourself and your own situation.

Chapter 1

WHAT'S It LIKE?

Each psilocybin journey is different, but here's my story

"I'm going to a cabin in the woods to do drugs with two people I've never met. And I've sent them a *bunch* of money."

Yep, when I say it out loud to friends or family, I hear how it sounds—like I've thrown caution into a tornado or that I'm attempting to live out a horror movie plot.

I pack my bag.

Bye forever

When I'm close to my destination, I pull over to text my husband, Jereme. I tell him I've made it and that I am about to drive up the mountain to the house.

He writes back, "Bye forever."

I shake my head and laugh. Then I put the SUV in drive and wind up a narrow, rutted road.

Jereme's only kidding; he knows I've done my research. But his message is symbolic. Perhaps he really is saying bye to what will eventually be the former me, someone who won't come back down this mountain.

I meet Gabriel Castillo and Bridgette Rivera at the remote cabin perched above the treetops. After giving me a few moments to shake off the drive, take in the view, and gulp the fresh air, Rivera "smudges me" by burning dried sage, a symbolic gesture to cleanse me of negative thoughts. She runs the smoke along my whole body, doing the soles of my feet one at a time, requiring an unexpected test of my balance, which feels off at such great heights. I pitch forward and grab the deck railing. When I laugh at myself, Rivera doesn't leave me hanging. She chuckles with me.

I instantly like her.

Let the ceremony begin

Castillo's guided meditation gives thanks to the east, south, west, and north, as well as the earth below that holds us and whatever may be above. I marvel at his words, considering that I'm about to embark on some serious navigation in my mind.

He invites me to take the medicine. I start with 1 gram of psilocybin that Castillo has ground into a powder and placed in a capsule. The strain is Cambodian, named for where it was found. It's known for its therapeutic journey, he tells me.

I lie beneath a weighted blanket on a cushioned floor mat and pull on an eye mask that obliterates all light. Castillo speaks a meditation into a microphone, his voice soothing but disembodied. On either side of me, both Castillo and Rivera play quartz singing bowls, bathing me in sound. Time passes, but I'm unaware of how much. I simply ease into a meditation. Eventually, Castillo invites me to ingest more medicine, so I sit up, grab the pill bottle he's placed beside my mat, and swallow another gram.

The whole experience is, at first, much like an amazing, meditative savasana, or corpse pose in yoga, traditionally included as a wind-down at the end of a session. But soon I enter something much deeper.

I am connected by threads of light to all the people I hold dear, located in different places. I visualize my friends and family as points on a map. My love for them flows along the threads to the points, and their love for me courses back. I think of fungi's wood wide web—that underground network that sends nourishment to plants in need in an ecosystem—and I'm in awe. Just imagine being able to feel the love, and everyone who loves you, as if all that love were surging on an electric circuit.

What a gift.

Their collective tenderness swaddles and cradles me. I'm safe inside it and allow my mind to take me places I have previously been afraid to go.

The mushroom acts as the Kool-Aid Man, crashing through walls I've carefully constructed to protect me. A loved one has wounded me repeatedly in recent years. And, if I'm being honest, the harm goes back much further. Time and distance have allowed a scarring over. But scarring leaves tougher skin to prevent future hurt. I've got a well of unconditional love for this person, one I keep covered. You do not leave such wells open—lest you fall in.

Now, in my mushroom meditation, I readily access my love, compassion, and empathy for them. I explore cherished, but bittersweet, memories of us. We're fishing. We're floating down the river. We're making up a secret wave for farmers we pass on the road.

Hurt cannot steal who I am or my love for this person or these memories. These things are mine. No one, no matter how much they gaslight me, can take them from me.

My eyes leak behind the mask. But here's the thing: I am not sad.

Castillo invites me to take more medicine. I like where I'm at and abstain. I still have another day to go deeper if I choose. And I will.

The mushroom crashes through another wall in my mind.

I access a memory of Fiver, our schipperke dog who passed away a year ago at age 11. We're running on a grassy back trail that's glittery with sunlight sneaking through the tree canopy. The memory becomes tangible, with the tug of his leash pulling me down his choice of snaking path. The moment is from the last time we were able to run together—just before he was diagnosed with congestive heart failure from a congenital valve defect. Jereme and I spent the next two years pouring all our energy into caring for Fiver, knowing the day would come when we'd have to let him go. But how do you let go of your living, breathing, panting, licking-your-face security blanket?

The mushroom takes me to the vet clinic. I do not fight it. I am holding Fiver for the last time. I kiss his forehead and inhale his scent to the bottom of my lungs, where it will imprint on my alveoli, where it will then flow into my heart to be pumped to my every cell. With him in my lap, I curl my body over his fluffy frame. He takes his last breath.

More tears wet the eye mask. But I am not sad. Fiver and I are together, and that will never change.

I've lost two friends recently and unexpectedly, one to an opioid overdose and one to natural causes when he collapsed on a street in New Orleans. I'd met both men in my twenties, and they became stalwart forces in my life. The losses of these beautiful humans have left me feeling as if a part of the past has also perished or been chopped off from my existence. In grieving them, I've also grieved the loss of the magical time when they first entered and became such a big part of my universe. When you lose pivotal people, you grieve them, of course. But you either knowingly or subconsciously also grieve a part of yourself because you are losing someone who witnessed different snapshots—iterations—of you. That time is still there, the mushroom shows me. It's still a part of me, and the *me* who lived that time is also still me. Ultimately, these men are with me and always will be. I am no longer severed from the past but threaded tightly to it.

Eventually, Castillo's gentle voice pulls me back into the room. Through guided meditation, he reacquaints me with my body and the space around me. I wiggle my fingers and toes, then my limbs. I've been so deep in my mind that it takes me a moment to adjust. I ask him how much time has passed. "Three hours," he says. My mouth drops open.

I grab my journal and scribble furiously. Castillo prepares dinner in the kitchen, giving me time to engage with my thoughts but making his presence known so that I feel safe if any heaviness crops up.

At dinner, I nibble at my food, even though the pesto pasta Castillo's prepared is delicious. My body is filled with warmth and love; I need no sustenance. But I'll be real: doing mushrooms can also temporarily kill your appetite. As we eat, Castillo and Rivera invite me to share about my experience. They are strangers, but somehow that fact makes it easier for me to tell them everything. I talk mostly about the one who has hurt me.

Before leaving for this trip—oh the pun!—I texted a friend who has experience with mushrooms. "I'm worried my trip will be all about——"

He wrote back immediately. "If it is, it will likely be healing." So far, he's correct.

That night, my brain is busy, but it doesn't spin like it often does before bed. It's busy exploring the opened spaces inside it. No longer is it a labyrinth with potential dead ends, scary dark corners, or covered wells. Instead, I can see where I am—as if on a windswept prairie in my home state, no skyscrapers blocking the view. I'm safe where I go.

I think about the one who has hurt me repeatedly and how that's impacted my life over the decades. I am being cryptic about who this person is; that is for their privacy. But this relationship represents such a core wound for me—one that has harmed me far more than I've ever realized or been willing to let myself understand before this moment.

I've kept others—but not all—at arm's length. I make new friends easily, and I love them without reserve. Even though I trust my friends, I don't always truly trust the friendship; I'm secretly waiting for the stick of dynamite to blow up the foundation.

The PSILOCYBIN HANDBOOK for Women

I'm not proud of the way I've let someone have so much power over me. But in this afterglow of the mushroom, I do not judge myself as I normally would. I recognize that the dynamics were put in place when I was a kid. I have empathy for the young girl I was. I am still her. I am proud of myself for showing her compassion and helping her grow instead of remaining stuck. I see a path forward toward healing and potential change. I can continue to love—from afar—this person who has hurt me, while protecting myself from further harm. Why do I love this person unconditionally? I've asked myself that question before. And a wise person once told me: "Because that's the definition of love—to love unconditionally." But also I know that the actions of the person who has hurt me are not born out of malice.

I lie awake for what seems like hours, exploring the reaches of my mind's expanse. Out my room's window, a lightning storm flickers, and I watch in awe until finally my brain is ready to rest.

The gauntlet

The next morning, Castillo prepares a breakfast spread. We eat, drink tea, and marvel at the view, our mountain peak appearing as if an island amid a sea of rolling fog. After breakfast, while we digest our food, Castillo leads us in another meditation, and we set our intentions for a new day with the mushroom and mind exploration. I'm ready when he invites me to ingest another gram of the Cambodian strain.

Rivera leads me in a restorative yoga session on the cabin's upper deck. We match each other with our inhales and exhales, relishing the scent of woodsmoke wafting up from the fire Castillo is building in a cauldron on the earth below us. My muscles loosen around my joints, and I feel a sense of readiness for what the day might bring.

We eventually find Castillo inside, brewing mushroom tea. He shows me his bag of B+ strain on the counter. Ensconced in plastic, the mushrooms are pristine. He hands both Rivera and me a mug, and we take our tea outside to the fire bowl.

While Castillo is my guide, Rivera is my trip sitter on this journey, a person who keeps an eye on you while you're tripping and helps ensure your safety and well-being. When I first contacted Castillo after finding his business Finally Detached online, we had an initial phone consultation followed by a video chat. I also filled out three forms he sent me. They inquired about my medical history and current medications, my mental state, my intentions for a psilocybin journey, and my history of trauma. Through these forms and various conversations, Castillo gleaned that I would be doing this trip alone, meaning without friends or my husband, and that— under the circumstances and my past experiences—I would feel safest with a female trip sitter present.

As my time with Rivera grows, so does the connection I feel with her, something that was instant upon us meeting. So I'm thrilled when she agrees to partake in the mushroom tea along with me. She's experienced with psilocybin, having done an 8-gram trip before, among others. (You can read her personal story with psilocybin in Chapter Four.) Having her by my side in this experience makes me feel like I have a sister taking me under her wing. And I'm completely at ease with Castillo by this point, as if he is somehow an old friend.

As a side note, I want to share why I chose these two lovely people— formerly strangers—to guide me through this new experience. I was researching options for a psilocybin retreat and came across Finally Detached. Castillo's program checked all my boxes. I could get to the location easily. He would provide the mushrooms. (FYI, this isn't always the case.) Castillo wasn't charging me extra for having a female present. Castillo's intake forms were extensive and put me at ease that he knew what he was doing and cared about my well-being. He provided me with several points of communication (phone calls and video chats) before the retreat. He also provided me with educational information to help me prepare. Plus, I had the option to be the only participant. The last point was important to me because other people's trip experiences—including the traumas they're processing—can impact your own. I knew I didn't want to participate in a large group setting, at least not for my first experience.

Castillo tosses bits of dried sage into the flames, then hands each of us pieces to toss in, as well. We again think of our intentions. When I let go of my piece, I visualize a sense of surrender to the experience, casting off any remaining doubt or fear. I'm ready for what the mushroom has to offer me today, whatever that may be. I inhale the burning sage, which again calls to mind the open range of my home state.

Rivera and I chat, cradled in our Adirondack chairs. We talk about our families of origin, a casual give-and-take of a conversation. When she next says something, I ask her if she can read my mind; I was just thinking the same thing. We laugh. Our talk tapers off, and we're both enjoying the view and the vibe. Castillo, who has been chilling in a hammock nearby, collects our empty mugs. "Do you want more?" he asks. We both say yes.

The sky releases an intermittent sprinkle. I tilt my head and relish the sensation of water hitting my face and becoming a part of me.

Have I ever felt anything so glorious?

I marvel at the texture of the moss on the tree in front of me and then on a rock near the firepit. It's such a green-green. And I am here in this moment to see it. I am euphoric. The mushroom has clearly taken effect.

"I give B+ an A+," I say.

Rivera laughs.

I move to the lower deck of the cabin and sit cross-legged, looking out at the mountains. They have a texture I've never noticed.

How cliché, I think. *Girl takes mushrooms and sees trees dance.*

But it's not a judgment. Then I'm crying. I am overwhelmed with gratitude for the people in my orbit—my parents, my friends, Jereme, everyone, even the person who has hurt me. I have gratitude for my life, my experiences. For Fiver.

Again, I am tightly connected to the past. I'm not necessarily visiting specific memories; it's more that I can feel the past. I can feel all that my 16-year relationship with Jereme is, from the moment of meeting him to now—not as a timeline, but rather as one complete essence that is still becoming all that it will be.

After leaving me alone with my euphoric tears for a bit, Rivera and Castillo invite me upstairs for lunch. I sit with Rivera facing out at the mountains. We get to know each other even more, and we marvel at the idea that the world is going on as usual while we're having this spectacular moment. Just as Castillo is about to join us, the wind picks up and the sky darkens and spits. We grab the dishes and food and dash inside, laughing. Castillo puts on a trippy video with a soundtrack to match.

Then things get weird.

The stool by the kitchen counter moves. The rocks on the fireplace pulsate. I look to my left. The couch exhales.

Can couches breathe?

I'm instantly anxious, but not because of the inanimate objects that have come to life. I'm entering a dark corner of my mind, one I've clearly been avoiding. The mushroom is taking me there, ready or not.

I am not surprised. It's a corner I hoped—albeit warily—to get into when I set my intentions for this trip. But now I want to hit "unsubscribe."

You cannot stop the ride on mushrooms though. Fight-or-flight mode kicks in, but I have nowhere to run. I'm tempted to flee to my cabin room and hide or find my phone and text Sara, a dear friend. Instead, I stay put on the breathing sectional. I channel Sara somehow, and she is in my mind with me, reaching out a figurative hand to guide me through this dark place.

"You are stronger than you think," I remember her telling me when my mom was diagnosed with cancer and I didn't know if I could face it all, even though I had to. I believed her then—because Sara had lost her dad and had been forced to realize her own strength. And I believe those words now. I surrender to the mushroom and let it pull me where it wants me to go.

In conversations with friends recently, I've brought up what I call "the gauntlet." This is the term I use for long stretches in life that are highly difficult and don't seem to have an end. We all must walk through them from time to time. For example, my dear friend McFeeny and his wife—parents of three young kids—are battling a long slog with her breast cancer diagnosis and ongoing treatment. Meanwhile, as a pulmonologist, he's just spent the entire pandemic treating the direst of patients. He lost his mom during the pandemic, as well. And my friend who recently collapsed in New Orleans was one of McFeeny's closest comrades. McFeeny is going through a major gauntlet for sure.

I face a gauntlet in the ensuing years. I don't know when it will come, but I know it's somewhere down the road. Like everyone eventually does, I will lose both of my parents. My mom, my absolute best friend, is now 80, and my dad is just a few years younger. The idea of losing them is hard to bear; it fills me with anxiety and makes my heart pound. It's a gauntlet that looms before me as this dark place with no light on the other side. I just picture deep, unending grief from one loss to the next and beyond. I also fear the behavior of the one who has hurt me. Will they inflict more pain on me at a time when I absolutely won't be able to take any more?

Now, the mushroom implores me to consider this feared gauntlet, to think about it, and to not look away. I obey.

The tears come.

Rivera and Castillo are nearby, quietly finishing their lunch. They do not rescue me from this dark place I've gone into. But I know they are there. I steal glances back at them to be sure.

My thoughts come fast then, showing me the difficult times or obstacles I've previously made it through—countless hospitalizations as a child and an adult, multiple endometriosis surgeries and eventually a hysterectomy, an ear surgery (to help with a hearing impairment) that left me bedridden with vertigo for weeks, a blood clot in my arm, my mom's back-to-back cancer diagnoses and treatments spanning two years, the untimely death of dear friends, the loss of Fiver, and a trauma I cannot bring myself to write about. These situations tick through my mind like a slideshow, but always I see the me who made it through every single one.

I sense the strength that Sara tells me I have. But I also sense her with me. A part of what helps me get through things is that I am not alone. I have people in my corner to lean on—people who have kindly been a balm for the pain of my core wound, people who have set me straight when a certain someone has gaslit me into caverns of self-doubt.

"The rain has stopped," Castillo tells me. "You can go back outside now."

I still need a few minutes and remain sitting there. Then finally, almost as if I've slipped into a hot bath, peace and relief flood my limbs. I untangle them from the sofa, which, thankfully, has stopped breathing. Just like that, I'm on a brighter side of my trip gauntlet. The literal and figurative storms have passed.

Castillo and Rivera head outside to revive our cauldron fire, leaving me to collect myself and join them when I'm ready. I find my phone in my room. Though the screen looks otherworldly to my tripping eyes and I can barely compose a text, I quickly message Sara—ever my beacon of light: "I love you, babe! Just had to say it."

Outside, Castillo asks me how I'm feeling. He's opening the door for an immediate integration session, a chance for me to talk through and process what I just experienced and to help me solidify my insights.

My thoughts come falling out of my mouth so fast that I am not sure I'm even making sense. I apologize for spewing words, but this is why I'm here. It's why they're here: to listen. I slow down. I tell them about my feared gauntlet and the trip gauntlet I just went through. I describe the anxiety. "It's the same feeling I've had in the last six miles of running a marathon," I say. This is when I doubt my capability to make it and I want to quit or ask someone else to step in. But no one else can do the work for me. (Not even superwoman Sara!) I've just got to put my head down and get through it, one stride at a time.

I see clearly now that I can get through life's gauntlets, too, even the one I fear the most. I will be okay. I have the tools. I've always had them. But I also have people in my life to support me. When my mom was going through chemo, my husband's friend, Josh, a guy who has become the brother I never had, took me aside. He'd lost both of his parents when he was in his twenties. He told me he could see the difficulty of the situation for me, and even though he'd been through something similar and that he's there for me, he said, "No one is living it exactly like you are right now." His words were a comfort because he saw me in that moment, and sometimes that's all you need for a strength boost. Even though I must walk—or run—through my own gauntlets, friends will be there to guide me the whole way while I do the hard work I've always done of getting myself through whatever it is. Lastly, I have no control over the one who has hurt me, but I do have control over how much power I give them. I can choose to give them none. I can choose to lean on the people who love me instead.

After I'm done speaking, Rivera tells me she fears losing her parents, too; it's a natural anxiety that's hard for her to see beyond. And Castillo tells us something so profound about death that I will never forget it. "When someone dies, you are no longer separate. That is when they become you."

I think of little Fiver and feel him in every cell.

After our talk, Castillo suggests a walk. So we hike to the bottom of the mountain and back up again, stopping to marvel at fungi along the way. We huff and sweat on our ascent until we reach our cabin on the peak and finally access a delightful breeze. The hike serves as a metaphor for having to climb out of the dark valley in the middle of my trip—my gauntlet. It also helps bring me back into my body after being so deep in my mind.

I once again take refuge on the lower deck and sit cross-legged to stare out at the mountains. My friends whom I've lost are with me. Fiver is with me. I am euphoric.

I was wrong. I will not come down the mountain and return to Jereme a new person. I will return knowing all that I am—feeling the essence of every chapter of my life—and open to all that I will become.

Chapter 2

GIVE ME the Microdose

What quick bits of info do I need as a newbie?

Babe, I got you. This chapter is a quick-hit Q&A section to answer some basic questions about psilocybin. The answers are shorties followed by suggestions on where to go next within the book for more info.

What is psilocybin (and psilocin) in a nutshell?

Psilocybin is a compound found in psychedelic fungi, meaning the mushrooms are mind altering or reality bending. *Psilocybe* is the genus name of more than 180 magic shroom species, some of which have multiple strains.[34] Psilocin is another compound found in magic mushrooms, but in smaller amounts than psilocybin. Additionally, after ingesting magic mushrooms, if that's your dosing method, your body converts psilocybin into psilocin.[35] That's your nutshell. But Chapter Three has more info.

What does psilocybin do?

Psychedelics change our awareness and perception of our immediate environment and ourselves, and they impact our thoughts and feelings. Psilocin and other magic mushroom compounds bind to serotonin receptors, especially in the prefrontal cortex[36]—the area of the brain that regulates mood and emotions. For this reason, magic mushrooms can alter thoughts, feelings, and more. In Chapter Three, you can read a monstrous section on what researchers say goes on in the brain and body during a trip.

What's it like to use magic mushrooms?

Magic mushrooms may elicit feelings of connectedness with others and nature, reduce awareness of the self or ego,[37] and enhance well-being—just to name a few effects. You may also experience more vivid memories. Magic mushrooms can distort your senses and impact your perception of space and time. The journey can be mystical, but in some cases, it may be intense or even disturbing. Some physical side effects may occur, as well. Many factors are at play when it comes to what you might feel. For more info on the potential effects of psilocybin, see Chapter Three. Stories of women's personal experiences with psilocybin are sprinkled throughout this book. Just visit the table of contents to find them.

Is psilocybin safe?

Psilocybin is one of the least toxic of recreational drugs.[38] It's on par with cannabis. However, many *other* mushrooms out there *are* extremely toxic and can kill you. Although psilocybin is considered generally safe, that phrase gets some major caveats. Chapter Five has robust safety info. But keep reading ...

Can I overdose on psilocybin?

The term "overdose" can get coupled with death because many people have died from overdosing on substances like opioids. Psilocybin can sometimes have unpleasant effects in the form of nausea or a challenging trip. But magic mushrooms aren't *generally* life-threatening. Again, you'll find safety considerations, some of them major, in Chapter Five.

Can I become addicted to psilocybin?

Psilocybin is not considered a physically addictive drug. Instead, it is being studied to potentially treat addiction.[39] You can read about that in Chapter Eleven.

Does psilocybin interact with any medications?

The short answer is: potentially. You can find the longer answer in the safety section in Chapter Five.

Who should not use psilocybin?

I'm no gatekeeper. Everyone must decide for themselves. But research is scant regarding the safety of psilocybin on a fetus when someone is pregnant or on a child when someone is breastfeeding/chestfeeding.[40] So while psilocybin use is *generally* not recommended under those circumstances, this topic deserves way more nuance than I can provide here. Chapter Eight is entirely dedicated to psilocybin and parenting. Additionally, for various reasons, you may wish to avoid using psilocybin while on certain medications or if you have certain underlying medical conditions. I provide more nuanced info on these topics in Chapter Five.

Is psilocybin legal and how do I get it?

I'm not your dealer! Just kidding. Psilocybin is legal in some places. The rest of the answer is more complicated than what can fit in an FAQ section. And the legal landscape of psychedelics is changing rapidly. I elaborate in Chapter Ten.

Does psilocybin show up on a drug test?

Psilocybin and psilocin end up in your pee. But not for long. Within 24 hours, they're undetectable.[41] Most magic mushroom compounds are actually excreted within a few hours of consumption.[42] Even if you were drug tested within a detectable window, most typical drug tests don't screen for psilocybin. The ones that do are special and expensive.

Alrighty! You've had your microdose. Now you're ready for a full info trip. You'll find that in Chapter Three. Or you can simply keep turning the pages ...

Chapter 3

GIVE ME the Full Trip

What are all the nitty-gritty details about psilocybin?

You want answers? I've got 'em. What follows are the potential effects of psilocybin on your body and brain. I can't help but think of that late '80s commercial. You know the one with the egg cracked into the frying pan and the subsequent sizzle? It had the tagline: "This is your brain on drugs. Any questions?" Well, after doing this research and trying psilocybin for myself, if I were to make a commercial about the brain on magic mushrooms, it would showcase a flower blooming. But you came here for a better explanation than that. So I present to you some of the neurobiology (mechanisms in the brain) and phenomenology (experiences during altered states of consciousness), plus the bodily side effects that may also occur during a trip.

I'm using the word *trip* here because in this chapter I'm not referring to microdosing, in which—although some mechanisms would occur—you wouldn't likely have noticeable psychedelic effects. (I cover dosing and microdosing in Chapter Ten.)

I go in depth on the effects because sometimes health journalism— especially that directed at women—tends to summarize and gloss over the specifics. I'm the kind of gal who asks "but why?" and "but how?" So I'm providing as much detail as possible.

What's the difference between psilocybin and psilocin?

Content about psychedelics often references psilocybin as the key compound in magic mushrooms. But psilocybin eventually becomes psilocin in your body. Psilocin is what becomes bioavailable and crosses from the bloodstream into the brain. Psilocin, then, is the active compound that produces the psychedelic effects. Therefore, psilocybin is a prodrug of psilocin.[43] For simplicity, I will mainly continue to reference psilocybin throughout this book. But first, I want to make clear the difference between psilocybin and psilocin.

Psilocybin—or *4-phosphoryloxy-N,N-dimethyltryptamine* as it's known chemically—is found in the *Psilocybe* genus, or what we simply call magic mushrooms. Psilocin is *4-hydroxy-N,N-dimethyltryptamine*. I mention the chemical names to illustrate what happens to psilocybin after you ingest magic mushrooms. Your stomach acids dephosphorylate, or metabolize, psilocybin into psilocin. Other parts of the digestive tract play a role, as well as the kidneys and the bloodstream.[44] When you look at the chemical names again, you can see that psilocybin becomes psilocin when the phosphate group is gone.

How long will the effects of psilocybin last?

Psilocybin's effects will kick in anywhere from 10 to 40 minutes, depending on how you consume magic mushrooms and whether you do so on an empty stomach. (On a full stomach, effects may take longer to appear.) Effects will last anywhere from three to six hours.[45]

What are psilocybin's effects on the brain?

First, let me be clear that researchers are still trying to figure out all of psilocybin's effects and exact mechanisms of action. Also, everyone's experience on magic mushrooms is different. That's in part because our brains differ in many aspects, including the sum of our experiences, traumas, memories, beliefs, and more. Plus, set and setting (covered in Chapter Ten) also impact a psilocybin experience.

As I dive into the science, I also want to acknowledge the magical aspect. How did the mushroom know exactly what I needed to learn during my trip? Somehow the mushroom allowed my mind to teach myself about the tools I have within me. Although some of what occurred can be explained by existing research, it still seems pretty magical to me, especially when we consider how meaningful psychedelic journeys can be.

Participants in psilocybin studies have repeatedly rated their experience on magic mushrooms as among the most meaningful in their lives.[46] That sense of meaning often correlates with having a mystical experience during a trip.[47] I discuss mysticism at the end of this brain section, because, weirdly, to understand more about mystical experiences, it helps to understand the mechanisms and phenomenology.

Of course, bad or challenging trips do happen. (See Chapter Ten.) But one thing of note is that in a 2016 study of nearly 2,000 psilocybin users surveyed about their most psychologically challenging trip, 84 percent said they benefited from the experience.[48]

Tryptamine alkaloids and serotonin

Both psilocybin and psilocin are tryptamine alkaloids. They are structural analogs to—meaning they are like or mimic—the neurotransmitter serotonin.[49] As a neurotransmitter, serotonin serves as a chemical messenger between nerve cells, not only in the brain but all over. It plays a role in digestion, body temperature, libido, cognition, and more. But one of serotonin's most well-known roles is regulating mood, specifically boosting it. Yay!

Psilocybin is a serotonin (5-hydroxytryptamine) 2A/1A receptor agonist. That means psilocybin binds to these serotonin receptors. (Psilocin has a higher binding ability than psilocybin—hence why it is the active metabolite.) The binding causes a signal transduction; it essentially changes your normal serotonin pathways.[50] Additionally, research suggests that receptor activation encourages the release of glutamate, an excitatory neurotransmitter that then increases neuronal activity in the brain's prefrontal cortex.

What do these changes do to the brain? I cover each of these aspects in detail, but in summary, psilocybin may help you process trauma in new ways, disrupt negative thought patterns, experience memories in a new light, access remote memories, transcend the boundary of time, feel more creative, feel more connected to others or the world at large, and gain a larger sense of empathy.

REBUS model

Researchers and neuroscientists have developed models for explaining or understanding what happens to our brains on psychedelics. One is the RElaxed Beliefs Under pSychedelics model, or REBUS and the anarchic brain.[51] It encompasses the free-energy principle.[52] And it involves the entropic brain hypothesis.[53] Robin Carhart-Harris, PhD, who heads the Centre for Psychedelic Research at Imperial College London, and theoretical neuroscientist Karl J. Friston, FMedSci, of the University College London, created REBUS.

As our lives unfold, the data our brains receive teach us about how the world works. We use that data to form our belief systems. By the time we're adults, our belief systems make our brains more constrained or inhibited than, say, when we were hopscotching on the recess playground back in the day. Our belief systems form a hierarchy, and during normal states of consciousness, the rigid "top-down" beliefs can prevent the flow of "bottom-up" information. Essentially, with that hierarchy in place, our adult belief systems can act like a domineering boss, preventing different perceptions from challenging them. However, psychedelics can relax that hierarchy to allow for bottom-up info to gain traction.[54]

How do our brains form this hierarchy in the first place? Our belief systems take shape over time through predictive coding. We predict a certain outcome, and then that outcome occurs again and again. When a surprise happens, it's a prediction error, according to the REBUS model. But, because of the uncertainty surprises create, our brains generally dislike prediction errors. This may be especially true if uncertainty has previously caused us harm, as in the case of trauma. Hence, our top-down beliefs may suppress any of those bottom-up perceptions.[55] Our belief systems can become so rigid that they try to prevent prediction errors from carrying any weight. We might even try to explain them away so that we can keep believing what we believe. That's why we can get stuck in certain thought patterns or behaviors that don't serve us, even when bottom-up info is trying to give us a helpful belief-system revision.

Consider an example. Fictional Kim was mauled by a fictional dog when she was a child. Understandably, Kim is terrified of dogs as an adult. Repeatedly dogs have barked at her when she's been out walking, jumped on her when she's been at friends' homes, and just all around continued to scare her. The belief that dogs are bad carries heavy weight for Kim. Then Kim's neighbor adopts a well-behaved golden retriever. This dog never barks. Goldie even sits at attention like a good boy when Kim passes his house. Aye, the surprise—the prediction error. This seemingly well-behaved dog is one exception to Kim's otherwise solid track record of encountering what she perceives as "bad" dogs. So the prediction error carries little weight, and it creates uncertainty. Kim's brain explains away Goldie's good behavior. *Perhaps he's just waiting for the right opportunity to attack,* she thinks. Kim still assumes this dog is inherently bad, and she wants nothing to do with Goldie. Her original rigid belief suppresses the prediction error.

Researchers theorize that our neurodynamics can be rigid and ordered in normal states of consciousness; they are less entropic. When we must think outside the box or be creative, our brains lean toward slightly more flexible and disorganized states; they are more entropic. Under psychedelics, however, the neurodynamics are quite entropic.[56] The REBUS model suggests that psychedelics allow us to excessively relax our predictive coding, and those rigid beliefs can then be reexamined and even revised.[57]

In fictional Kim's case, the rigid belief is that all dogs are bad—no exceptions. Remember, for her, that's the belief that normally carries all the weight and suppresses any prediction errors. But with a more entropic brain on psilocybin,[58] that prediction error she encountered (Goldie is actually well-behaved! What?) gains more weight and may even usurp the heavy belief (all dogs are bad) by gaining traction in her belief hierarchy. Perhaps Kim will even work her way up to giving good-boy Goldie an ear scratch.

I'm not suggesting psilocybin will help people get over their fear of dogs. I'm simply using this as an easy-to-understand example of how our belief systems can get locked in and how revision can be helpful.

You'll find more on the REBUS model in the *ego death* section, just ahead.

Neuroplasticity and BDNF

Further showcasing the potential for mind expansion and personal growth is the preclinical evidence that psilocybin promotes neuroplasticity, the brain's ability to change and adapt.[59]

"We all have neuroplasticity to some degree," explains Abigail Calder, MSc, "although it's highest in children and young adults." Learning, forming memories, and adapting to our environment all require neuroplasticity. "It's also needed to heal the brain," Calder adds. "A classic example of neuroplasticity is that when a stroke destroys some brain cells, other cells learn to take over some of their function."

Calder is a doctoral researcher at the University Center for Psychiatric Research at the University of Fribourg in Switzerland. She recently coauthored a paper published in the journal *Neuropsychopharmacology* on psychedelic-induced neuroplasticity,[60] so I pepper her with questions via email, and she kindly writes back to explain more.

In her paper, Calder notes the theory that psychedelics are "psychoplastogens." David Olson, PhD, of UC Davis, coined the term.[61] "He uses it to refer to small molecules that rapidly and lastingly enhance neuroplasticity after a single dose," Calder explains. "Most psychedelics do this, including ketamine and MDMA." (MDMA is also commonly referred to as "ecstasy" or "molly.")

During a period of enhanced neuroplasticity, such as what would occur during and after a psilocybin journey, your brain is more pliable. "If you think of your brain as a sword on a blacksmith's anvil," she adds, "more neuroplasticity means your brain is hotter and thus more able to be re-shaped. So anything that happens during this time is more likely to have a lasting effect on you, limited by the specific brain regions affected."

Calder's lab is currently collecting data on how long psychedelics enhance neuroplasticity in humans. In mice, she notes, it's three to five days. "Things that happen during this period may have greater power to shape your brain than they otherwise would," Calder continues, "including the trip itself."

Some benefits of neuroplasticity last beyond the period of enhancement. "After the window of plasticity closes," Calder explains, "studies also show that the new dendrites formed during that time mostly persist. So even after neuroplasticity returns to normal, you get to keep your new connections." But not necessarily forever. "The new connections are still only made of brain tissue, not titanium," Calder adds. "She who does not use them will lose them. The lasting effect ultimately depends on your choice to uphold—or overwrite—any changes that occurred."

Psilocybin and other psychedelics appear to boost neuroplasticity via their 5-HT_{2A} receptor action. "They activate this receptor in a unique way," Calder says, "and appear to trigger a positive feedback loop, which promotes neuroplasticity even after the drug has left the body." The 5-HT$_{2A}$ receptor activation enhances the expression of brain-derived neurotropic factor (BDNF). "'Neurotrophic' means that it essentially helps the brain grow," Calder says. "In neurons, BDNF promotes the growth of new dendrites (neuronal branches which connect to other cells) and new synapses (connections between cells)." BDNF also encourages the growth of new neurons (neurogenesis). But this only occurs in select brain regions. "Most psychedelics don't seem to affect neurogenesis so far," Calder adds. In the positive feedback loop, "BDNF acts on its endogenous receptor (TrkB, pronounced 'track bee')," she explains, "which promotes both the growth of dendrites and the strengthening of synapses. TrkB promotes synaptic strength by enhancing the expression of AMPA receptors, which in turn enhance BDNF expression, now without the psychedelic drug being necessary— that's the feedback loop. Meanwhile, TrkB activity also promotes the growth of dendrites, partially via a protein called mTOR." I don't want to digress too much, but in case you are wondering, AMPA receptors (AMPA being short for *a-amino-3-hydroxy-5-methyl-4-isoxazolepropionic acid*) control most fast excitatory synaptic transmission in the central nervous system.

Magic mushrooms increase BDNF in mice.[62] "We don't know a lot about psilocybin's effects on BDNF in humans," Calder says. That's because studies so far have produced mixed results. Complicating the research is the fact that, in humans, BDNF can only be measured in peripheral blood. "It's not clear at all that BDNF in the blood reflects BDNF in the brain," Calder explains. "What's [clearer] is that psilocybin promotes the growth of dendrites and synapses. Perhaps this also involves promoting BDNF, but more research is needed."

Psilocybin's mechanisms of action on the brain are what boost neuroplasticity; it's not the trip itself. "Cells in a culture dish also show enhanced neuroplasticity after psychedelics," Calder notes, "and they are probably not having any experience at all! But that doesn't mean that the trip is not important. The trip experience is taking place within a highly plastic brain. This means that the experiences that people have during and shortly after the trip may have more lasting effects than experiences had at other times."

Now that we have a handle on some of the potential mechanisms, let's get into the specifics of what you might experience during a psilocybin trip.

Ego death: psilocybin's impact on the default mode network

Depending on the dose, psilocybin can cause what's called "ego death" or "ego dissolution."[63] That's because it impacts the default mode network. The DMN is a network of brain regions that work together. The network is suppressed when you're focused on the external world, like replying to emails, giving a presentation, scrolling through social media, filing your taxes, etc. Instead, the DMN is all about your internal world and is active when your mind is free to wander. It's often active when you're doing a routine task, like taking a shower or folding laundry. Maybe you're wondering about your future or mulling over memories—doing what's called "mental time travel."[64] Maybe you're trying to understand yourself better. Ultimately, the DMN is concerned with your narrative self and how *you* see *you* in the world.

In childhood and adolescence, your DMN is sparsely connected, but it undergoes rapid architectural changes as you develop your sense of self.[65] The DMN becomes even more integrated as you continue to solidify whom you are in adulthood.[66] Of course, not all the ways in which we view ourselves are helpful to us. (Lookin' at you, inner critic!) Our DMN can become so rigid that we have a hard time interrupting those communication pathways our brain has built. Remember the REBUS model, which suggests we can have heavy belief systems that suppress new input.[67]

Magic mushrooms and some other psychedelics, researchers theorize, "decouple" or unplug the DMN from the medial temporal lobe. The MTL, important for memory and the self, includes the hippocampus, the parahippocampal regions, and the amygdala, among other parts of the brain. Psilocybin potentially causes a decrease in connectivity between brain hemispheres, also affecting the MTL.[68] These changes in connectivity cause a temporary loss of identity and ego in general.[69] There's even an acronym for this whole concept: DIED (drug-induced ego dissolution).[70]

Hold the phone! That sounds terrifying—and it can be. But, depending on dose, you may not experience a full-on ego murder during your trip, just some beneficial elements of reduced ego that I explain in this chapter.

You might be wondering how losing your identity—either full or partially—can be useful. The researchers who came up with the REBUS model provide a concept to help us understand.[71] Imagine dropping a heavy ball (think of this as a different perception) on a frozen pond (your brain's belief system). The ball doesn't do much, if anything, to the rigid surface. Now imagine dropping that same ball on a thawed pond. The ball enters the water with a splash and causes a ripple effect. While conditions like depression can cause a more frozen belief system that doesn't allow for different input, psychedelics may thaw that rigid system and allow for alternate perceptions and subsequent change.

Maybe your sense of self is cluttered with outdated beliefs or thought patterns that are holding you back from being open in your friendships, from leaving an unhealthy relationship, from seeking a new job—from whatever it is. Ego death may serve as a sense-of-self reboot by changing the belief hierarchy and disarming defenses[72]—that frozen belief system.

Here's a simple example: I get together with a group of female friends frequently. We've all talked about how we often wake up the next day after hanging out and wonder if we've offended the others, talked too much, or otherwise said something stupid. We collectively agree these worries are silly; none of us judge each other or ever wake up mad at someone else in the group. On the contrary, we're always grateful for the time we spent together, and aside from our own self-doubts, we feel renewed from our gathering. Yet my friends and I can individually get stuck in this negative thought pattern of thinking we somehow effed up.

Why? It's likely due to some aspect of overactivity or changes in connectivity in the DMN. Differences in connectivity are present in some mental health conditions, including anxiety, obsessive-compulsive disorder, and more.[73] That's not to say that if you have this same thought pattern I just described—or a different one—that you have these diagnoses. Anyone can simply battle negative ideas about themselves from time to time. That's part of being human. Psilocybin may be able to help you break negative patterns that are interfering with your life. For example, on magic mushrooms, I could see that these friends care about me and enjoy my presence, and I've held on to that belief since my trip.

Fear extinction: psilocybin's effects on the limbic system

During a trip, you may be able to revisit a trauma and process it without the memory's associated panic and fear.[74] That's because psilocybin impacts the limbic system, which includes the amygdala, your fear center. The amygdala—or amygdalae since we have two—plays a key role in how we process and react to both positive and negative emotions in relation to stimuli. The amygdala also helps encode emotional memories. If you've experienced a traumatic event, your amygdala has cataloged and tagged it. And that's why negative stimuli—scents, sounds, images, sensations—that remind your brain of that traumatic event can elicit a fresh panic or fear response. Psilocybin has been shown to boost mood, but it also reduces our processing of negative stimuli and reduces amygdala reactivity to perceived threats.[75] Evidence in animal studies shows that psilocybin causes "fear extinction."[76] Some of these impacts may last beyond your trip. Of course, fear and anxiety can also be present during a trip.[77] (See Chapter Ten.)

Autobiographical memory: gaining new insight

Despite ego dissolution, you can still access autobiographical memories—potentially even ones you avoid or have forgotten—and you may even experience them more vividly.[78] The exact effects of psilocybin on memory are still being studied. Brain images of people on magic mushrooms show changes in brainwave synchronization between the parahippocampal cortex and the retrosplenial cortex—which is a memory gateway to the DMN—and parts of the prefrontal cortex. Some researchers theorize that these alterations allow for an enhanced reprocessing of autobiographical memories, offering us new insight.[79] With the sense of self zoomed out and less activation of the amygdala telling us about all the emotional tags we associated with a memory, perhaps we're able to view autobiographical memories with fresh perspective and process them differently.

Helioscope effect: revisiting trauma without getting "burned"

Calder's coauthor, Gregor Hasler, MD, also of the University of Fribourg, created a metaphor for the phenomenon of viewing painful events from a safe distance: the "helioscope effect."[80] Calder explains Hasler's concept: "A helioscope is a special telescope that you can use to view the sun, which is normally too painful to gaze at." Psychedelics can act like a helioscope for viewing the difficult things life has thrown or spit at us. "They allow people to process things that are normally too painful to think about," Calder says. MDMA is particularly known for this effect. "In trauma therapy, for example," Calder explains, "MDMA can make traumatic experiences psychologically safer to process so that people can work through them without being 'burned' by their heat or overwhelmed." Such processing may lower the risk of re-traumatization when compared to other methods, like talk therapy alone. But more than that, Calder adds, psychedelics' helioscope effect occurs inside a brain in which neuroplasticity has just been boosted. "This means that the trauma processing people undergo on psychedelics," she notes, "is more likely to [have] a lasting effect than trauma processing done without enhanced neuroplasticity."

However, Calder shares a caution. "A key component of this is also that the psychedelic drug must be allowed to 'choose' the content of the trip without much interference," she says. "Left to their own devices, psychedelics in a therapeutic setting naturally bring up problems, memories, and emotions that may be painful, but are not usually overwhelming." In other words, the helioscope effect unfolds naturally and doesn't require pressure. "If there is a therapist pushing someone to re-experience a particular trauma on psychedelics and the patient is not ready," Calder says, "that therapist could actually be undermining the helioscope effect." (You can read about some important safety considerations regarding psychedelic-assisted therapy in Chapters Five and Six.) "The helioscope effect thus has to be supported by the right setting," Calder adds, "and the right amount of zipping it while the drug is working."

Oceanic boundlessness: a sense of unity

The zoomed-out sense of self brought on by ego death may help in other ways too. Our sense of self can be isolating, simply because we think of ourselves as individuals going through our own individual challenges. Taking ego out of the equation helps to dissolve the boundary of self and other. You may experience a sense of "oceanic boundlessness."[81] Oceanic boundlessness is a term derived from a conversation between Sigmund Freud and Romain Rolland, a

French mystic.[82] The term ultimately means having no bounds. And the sensation can feel like a profound connectedness with the rest of the world, the people you love, those in your immediate presence, the flora and fauna, or even inanimate objects.

Theory of mind: an empathy boost

The DMN is also important for "theory of mind."[83] Theory of mind involves our ability to understand others, including empathizing and interpreting someone else's emotions and predicting their behavior. Psilocybin may increase empathic functioning.[84] Researchers aren't sure as to the exact mechanisms yet, but one hypothesis is that a decreased focus on the self and an increase in sense of unity help us find an equilibrium that may up empathy. Likewise, psilocybin increases openness, which may also provide an empathy boost.[85] Maybe as a unifier, psilocybin simply encourages us to stop seeing each other as *other*.

"It's maybe serving as a bridge for some people," says Bea Chan. Chan is the cofounder of Sisters in Psychedelics (SIP),[86] a resource you can read about in Chapter Six. She's referring to all psychedelics. "I think most of them are heart openers," she adds. "You can put yourself in the shoes of the other person and feel what they're carrying and see things from their perspective." SIP hosts integration circles for people to help process their psychedelic experiences. Chan notes that in these circles, people often discuss an empathy boost and how it helped. "I've definitely heard a lot about patching up their relationship to their families," she says.

Time isn't real: psilocybin's impact on time perception

After my first trip, I texted my husband and said, "Time isn't real." You, too, might have some wonky experiences regarding time while on psilocybin. One is that your concept of time may be impaired. And another is that you might feel you have transcended the construct of time entirely. These experiences might be somewhat related to each other.

Research shows that many people, while on magic mushrooms, experience time as moving a bit slower.[87] That's likely because of psilocybin's impact on our serotonin receptors, which help us discern longer time intervals.[88] But more research is needed. Transcendence of time could mean many things, such as a feeling of existence beyond this earthly realm or the ability to time travel mentally.[89] The former might be related to oceanic boundlessness. If you feel connected to the universe at large, time may no longer be a boundary for you. And with the potential ability to access remote memories or to envision your future, you may feel like you've broken through a time boundary.

Enhanced creativity: a more flexible mind

While under the influence of psilocybin, you may experience heightened creativity, and the benefits may last beyond your trip.[90] Some studies show that psilocybin decreases the brain's rigidity that we're used to in normal states of consciousness and encourages a more flexible state.[91] These changes could benefit us creatively, but more research is needed to understand the exact mechanisms and potential.

Normally our brains have highly organized activity within the brain's three resting-state networks (including the DMN). But under psilocybin, research shows we experience a relaxation of all that law and order.[92] At the same time, we experience an increased coupling between resting-state networks that normally don't couple. Some connectivity changes are present up to one month post-dose.[93]

Mystical experiences: the awe-factor

Mystical experiences seem to play a central role in meaningful and life-changing psychedelic journeys.[94] But they occur outside of psychedelic journeys as well, often in a spiritual, religious, or meditative context. Under the influence of psilocybin, a mystical experience often features aspects of ego dissolution and oceanic boundlessness.[95]

In a small 2008 double-blind study, researchers examined mystical-type experiences in participants who tried psilocybin for the first time. The volunteers engaged in two or three therapy sessions; in these sessions, they were unaware of whether they were receiving a moderate or high dose of psilocybin, a low dose, or an inactive placebo. The researchers followed up with the study participants 14 months later. Of the 36 participants, 58 percent rated their psilocybin experience as one of the five most meaningful in their lives, while 67 percent said it was their most spiritually significant. More than half (58 percent) met criteria for a full-blown mystical experience.[96]

The researchers used the Pahnke-Richards Mystical Experience Questionnaire to assess the participants' trips. The criteria of a mystical trip included experiencing the following: a sense of unity with all or a pure awareness, transcendence of space and time, difficulty describing the experience, a sense of awe, knowledge of "ultimate reality," and an intensely positive mood. Also at follow-up, 64 percent of participants reported that psilocybin had increased their life satisfaction or overall well-being, and 61 percent said it was a catalyst for positive behavioral change.

What are psilocybin's effects on the body?

You may experience some physical side effects while on psilocybin. Most are a result of psilocybin's impact on serotonin receptors and changes to the autonomic nervous system, which regulates our involuntary bodily processes, like heart rate.

Your pupils will likely become dilated.[97] You may experience enhanced perceptions, visual distortions, or even hallucinations. Your senses may feel connected in what's known as synesthesia.[98] You might notice a loss of coordination,[99] or you may feel dizzy.[100] Your blood pressure might become elevated,[101] and your heart rate may speed up.[102] You may also notice a rise in body temperature. You might feel nauseated or have a change in appetite. After a trip, you may also notice temporary changes in sleep,[103] such as a disruption in your ability to nod off. More research is needed on these potential side effects, but here's a brief explanation of each.

Eye and vision changes

Serotonin agonists, such as psilocybin, can impact the iris dilator, causing the pupils to become dilated.[104] During a trip, you may also see color more vividly or in different ways. Researchers theorize that changes in color perception are a result of uninhibited signaling and increased neural plasticity. People who experience color blindness have even reported improved color perception following psychedelic use.[105]

Visual distortions are a characteristic of many psilocybin trips. Distortions may include seeing a host of geometric patterns (such as a honeycomb, cobweb, tunnel, or spiral), experiencing changes in the way we perceive object borders, and noticing items that appear to be breathing. Researchers attribute these hallucinations to abnormal activation of cortical neurons.[106] People also experience hallucinations of entities or beings or bodily distortions of themselves while on psilocybin. Although more research is needed, scientists attribute these to the reduced organization and connectivity of brain networks.[107]

Synesthesia

Also, likely because of changes in brain region connectivity and changes in neurotransmitters, is synesthesia.[108] Synesthesia is when you experience one or more senses through another. During a psilocybin journey, you might see yellow when you hear a bird's song, for example. Or you might taste a sound or a word, even though you haven't eaten a thing.

Loss of coordination or feeling dizzy

While on psilocybin, you might not be as graceful as you normally are. This may occur for a few reasons. One, our serotonergic pathways play a role in how we move.[109] As a serotonin receptor agonist, psilocybin temporarily alters these pathways. And two, your visual perception may also be distorted as previously described. So that coffee table may seem to jump out at you. Oops.

Cardiovascular and body temperature changes

Psilocybin may increase blood pressure and heart rate, and in a related side effect, may increase body temperature. These changes are related to the compound's effects on the autonomic nervous system. The autonomic nervous system has three divisions. One is the sympathetic nervous system, which controls our fight-or-flight response. Psilocybin can cause sympathetic nervous system arousal.[110] For this reason, you should consider whether you have an underlying cardiovascular condition before using psilocybin or other psychedelics. (See Chapter Five.)

Gastrointestinal symptoms

One of the most annoying potential side effects of magic mushrooms is nausea. Research is still out on what exactly causes the nausea, but evidence points to a possibility. First, mushroom cell walls, unless cooked,[111] consist of chitin, a hard-to-digest compound.[112] Enzymatic breakdown of chitin in your stomach may give rise to queasiness via an inflammatory response.[113]

However, some people still experience nausea, even if they opt for another method of ingesting, such as a tea. We also have serotonin receptors in the gut; approximately 95 percent of our serotonin is found there.[114] And our guts and brains are connected via a gut-brain axis. Psychedelics can cause smooth muscle contraction in the gastrointestinal tract. All these factors may play a role in nausea. Plus, you may have a lot going on in the brain during a psychedelic trip. Therefore, the impact on the gut-brain connection, which involves the autonomic nervous system (both the fight-or-flight and the rest-and-digest responses), may also induce an upset stomach.[115] In normal states of consciousness, you may have felt sick to your stomach when receiving bad news, for example. That's the autonomic nervous system doing its thing. Since the gut-brain axis is affected, you may also notice a change in appetite during or after your psilocybin experience.

Changes in sleep

Likely you won't sleep during a magic mushroom trip, but you may also have delayed sleep after one. More research is needed on how psilocybin affects sleep. But research in rodents shows delayed rapid-eye movement (REM) sleep and reduced non-REM sleep up to three hours after a dose.[116] Long-term disruption to the sleep-wake cycle does not appear to be a concern, however.

As you can see, a lot happens in the brain and body overall during a psilocybin trip. If you're wondering how these effects all translate to potential benefits (or not) for specific conditions, Chapter Eleven has all the details on the research so far.

Chapter 4

BRIDGETTE'S STORY

Healing from disordered eating

If you read Chapter One, you'll recall the name Bridgette Rivera. Rivera was my trip sitter. In talking with her during my magic mushroom retreat, I learned her personal story with psilocybin and how it helped her recover from disordered eating and heal from childhood trauma. After the retreat, I asked if I could interview her for this book to provide insight to others.

"I want to continue to live in this highest vibration, which is love," Rivera tells me when we're on the phone about a month after first meeting. "Psilocybin has gotten me so connected with the source—I feel I am that. I'm healing myself every day without even taking the medicine. It's in my DNA now. It's just a part of me forever. And it's the most beautiful thing."

An eating disorder is born

Rivera wasn't always so at peace with life. In her teen years, she was part of a dance company. "Dance was my life," she says. But a dance instructor who placed a scale in the dance room threatened everything. Before every session, Rivera's instructor weighed her students and logged the numbers. "I was the heaviest in the class," Rivera recalls. "I was put on a probation. And that probational period—that's when it started for me. I had to do something."

After three hours of dance classes, Rivera would go home, layer trash bags over a jumpsuit, and ride her stationary bike for hours. She also changed her eating habits, opting for a small salad, while everyone else in the family ate a full meal. "They had no awareness of the level of desperation I was living," she says of her parents.

Two weeks into her new routine, everything changed for Rivera at the dance company. "I went into class," Rivera says, "and the teacher turned around and she stopped the music. She pulled me up to the front of the class. She said, 'Everybody, look at Bridgette … I don't know what you're doing, Bridgette, but you keep doing it.'"

From then on, the instructor placed Rivera at the front of the line and gave her the parts she wanted. And Rivera kept doing what she had been told to do: overexercise and starve herself.

At 18, Rivera became pregnant with her son, Gabriel Castillo. Her pregnancy temporarily halted the disordered eating. "The nine months I was pregnant," she recalls, "I ate. I ate because I knew it was not just about me." But the reprieve was temporary.

Going from living with her parents to living with and being married to the father of her child, while also being a mother, left Rivera no chance to cultivate her independence and find her true self. "I walked out of a home that was kind of structured," she says. "It was very controlling. My dad's way or the highway." She describes her mom, however, as being submissive. "I walked into a relationship that was very much similar to that." She clarifies that her marriage was not abusive, but instead, in retrospect, was supportive. The issue, she says, was rooted in her own submissiveness, a dynamic she learned from her parents. "I had the opportunity to step up and speak," she says, "but I just never took it on."

Nevertheless, she says she felt a lack of power over her own life. Rivera is clear that a big part of that feeling of a loss of control was rooted in childhood trauma and was not solely about her romantic relationship or her upbringing—taken together, though, all aspects contributed. Her weight, however, was something she could control. She continued to starve herself, and she took up running. Plus, she became addicted to saunas. Rivera says she particularly engaged in these tactics when a feeling, like anger, triggered her. "It kind of just numbed it for a little bit," she explains.

The mushroom flips the switch

Eventually Rivera's marriage ended in divorce. Meanwhile, Castillo became an adult and went off to college, where he embarked on a journey of self-discovery. He sent his mom books and affirmations to help her. Later, with Castillo's guidance, Rivera elected to try psilocybin.

She describes her first journey on magic mushrooms as "heart opening." She tells me of a source or an energy or vibration that guided her, giving her a sense that she was not alone. "It was as if I was peeking through different aspects of my life," she explains. "It was showing me these visions and past experiences. I was able to see all the traumas pop up." But in many instances, she was viewing her memories from the perspective of someone else who had also been present. Rivera says that seeing things from the perspective of others encouraged empathy for those who had hurt her and that she was able to lean into forgiveness.

That journey prompted her to continue working with magic mushrooms. "I dug deep," Rivera says. "I spent the last five years just doing the work." She describes subsequent psilocybin journeys as peeling back layers of consciousness like peeling those of an onion. Now, in everyday life, when she thinks about her life's traumas, they are just thoughts. "There's no ache in my heart," she explains. "There's no pit in my stomach."

In one particularly deep journey, Rivera ingested about 8 grams of B+ strain in tea. She describes lasers of sunlight in a webbing emanating from everything, including the trees, rocks, grass, and from herself and Castillo, who was guiding her journey. "I was in amazement that I was seeing the vibration of the energy of everything," she recalls.

As for the eating disorder, she says it disappeared like the flip of a switch. "[The mushroom] showed me who I was and who I am," she explains. But also, psilocybin taught her that she is more than herself. "I am you, I am my son, I am everyone," she tells me. That realization increased her compassion for herself and her capacity for self-love. "I had to forgive myself," she adds. "And with that forgiveness was the switch."

Now, the eating disorder is not a part of her life. "If it is there," she says, "it is there simply because I have the awareness that I want to help others with it." She describes herself as having a healthy relationship with food now. "If I'm hungry," she says, "I'll listen. And I really listen to what I want." She enjoys cooking and no longer thinks about irrelevant numbers on a scale.

Chapter 5

SAFETY FIRST

I'm a safety gal. What are the concerns?

I'm 100 percent a safety gal. So I'm here for you on this. Psychedelic researchers generally report psilocybin to be safe and as having the "most favourable [sic] safety profile" of all psychedelic drugs.[117] As with everything considered safe (lookin' at you, scissors, laundry pods, bicycles), there are some caveats. And some of them are big caveats. When we talk about a psychedelic as generally safe, offer only a mini disclaimer about the parts that might not be safe, and then shine the spotlight on all the potential good points, that does a disservice to everyone.

In the case of psilocybin, some safety considerations apply to underlying medical conditions and related medications, which I cover in this chapter. But we still have a lot of stuff to learn. Additionally, in some cases, people have put themselves or others at risk of physical harm during a challenging trip.[118] Plus, *major* safety concerns exist surrounding all psychedelics and abuses of power. Some therapists, guides, and shamans have abused their clients while those clients have been in their care on and off psychedelics.[119] (See Chapter Six.)

Is psilocybin considered safe? And are there psilocybin-associated deaths?

A 2021 systematic research review looked at 52 psilocybin clinical trials. None reported serious adverse events.[120] However, 25 did not directly report on safety. Additionally—according to the Global Drug Survey 2021—of people who reported using magic mushrooms in the last 12 months, only 0.02 percent sought emergency medical treatment for any negative experiences.[121] That does not mean that negative experiences aren't happening. Bad trips and unpleasant side effects do occur.

Although overdose deaths from psilocybin aren't really a thing, I do want to make note of two deaths associated with psilocybin that we know about. In one instance, a 24-year-old woman went into cardiac arrest after ingesting magic mushrooms a few hours prior.[122] She had received a heart transplant a decade before. In another case, a 74-year-old man's heart stopped within an hour after he ingested psilocybin. In episode 8 of *New York* magazine's podcast *Cover Story: Power Trip*, Lily Kay Ross, PhD, discusses this incident.[123] While the autopsy originally noted psilocybin as the probable cause, the coroner later attributed the death to the man's heart condition.[124] But there's more to the story, and that's why I encourage you to listen to the show. Other associated deaths may have occurred that aren't reported in literature. But again, psilocybin is reported to have a low toxicity.[125]

What do I need to know about my drug supply?

Psilocybin may have a low toxicity, but deaths from unintentionally ingesting poisonous mushrooms do occur. The National Poison Data System keeps track of such cases in the United States; it recorded 52 fatalities and 704 incidents of major harm from toxicity from 1999 to 2016.[126] I don't recommend mushroom hunting for psilocybin.

Additionally, not everything you purchase is what it seems. It's worth checking to ensure that what you're planning to ingest is indeed psilocybin and nothing unexpected—like additional chemicals or drugs you don't want to ingest.

The Fireside Project, a nonprofit organization that focuses on psychedelic peer support, safety, and awareness, recommends testing your supply.[127] You can buy testing supplies online.

What do I need to know about psilocybin and underlying conditions?

I'm a lady with a litany of underlying health conditions, so I researched this topic thoroughly before trying psilocybin, and I'm providing you with that info here. I'm also adding the disclaimer that you should talk to your healthcare provider. However, not all physicians will be on board with recreational or therapeutic use of psilocybin, even if you're as healthy as the healthiest of horses and take zero medications. I'm not encouraging anyone to ignore their doctor's advice. I am encouraging you to do your research, employ common sense, and weigh the risks and benefits that apply to your unique situation. Ultimately, you must make your own decisions, and in no way should this chapter be construed as medical advice. I'm not a doctor.

Certain underlying conditions generally preclude someone from participating in a psilocybin clinical trial.[128] I'm sharing that info with you here so that you can make informed decisions about your health when it comes to magic mushrooms. If you have one of the underlying conditions listed in this chapter, you may wish to exercise certain cautions, use under medical supervision only, or avoid psilocybin altogether.

The clinical trial exclusion info does raise an issue regarding psychedelic studies, however. Psilocybin and other psychedelics have shown evidence of efficacy as therapeutics to ease symptoms of various conditions. But if trials are excluding entire groups of people, say those with schizophrenia, how will we know how psilocybin affects those with schizophrenia?[129] Clinical trials do, in some cases, enroll populations that are normally excluded, especially if the clinical trial is investigating the effects of psilocybin in that population, such as how magic mushrooms affect those with borderline personality disorder.[130] Other studies survey specific populations to learn more before considering additional research.

Again, you must make the best decision for you after weighing all benefits and risks. For example, randomized clinical trials now show that psilocybin may help with treatment-resistant depression.[131] Theoretically, someone may benefit from psilocybin's therapeutic potential despite having an underlying condition that traditionally excludes them from participating in a clinical trial. Does that mean they cannot try psilocybin to treat their depression? I can't provide an answer for that person's unique situation. The questions remain: If psilocybin might improve their quality of life, which could then improve their overall health, do the benefits outweigh any potential risks? And can that person try psilocybin in a way that reduces those risks, such as under medical supervision? As the research stands now, we don't have all the answers to those questions. All I can do in this book is provide you with the list of clinical trial exclusion data and why those underlying conditions are typically excluded.

Generally, cardiovascular conditions, liver conditions, seizure conditions, diabetes, some mental health conditions, and pregnancy or breastfeeding/chestfeeding prevent people from inclusion in psilocybin-specific studies. You can read about each of these topics in their individual sections. (However, you can find robust info on pregnancy or breastfeeding/chestfeeding—plus other topics surrounding psilocybin and parenting—in Chapter Eight.)

Cardiovascular conditions

I noted in the section on psilocybin's effects on the body and brain that magic mushrooms can elevate blood pressure and heart rate.[132] For these reasons, people with underlying heart conditions are not eligible for clinical trials. Heart conditions include, but are not limited to, uncontrolled high blood pressure, congestive heart failure, coronary artery disease, congenital heart defects, artificial heart valves, a history of stroke or heart attack, cardiac hypertrophy, heart arrhythmias, tachycardia, electrocardiographic abnormalities, etc.

Diabetes

People with insulin-dependent or uncontrolled diabetes are also generally excluded from psilocybin clinical trials. I cannot find specific research on what, if any, impact psilocybin itself has on blood sugar. But all the body and brain impacts present during a trip could cause glucose changes. Anecdotal reports online point to potential problems with low blood sugar during a trip. Many people start their magic mushroom journey on an empty stomach, which could be a factor or compound the issue. And reactive hypoglycemia (a blood-sugar crash after eating—usually within four hours) could also be at play, depending on multiple factors. Keep in mind that during a trip, you're in an altered state of mind, which could have implications for your usual chronic disease care. The bottom line is that tripping could have impacts on blood sugar and diabetes management, as it could for the management of any condition.

Liver conditions

Having liver impairment or liver disease also prevents someone from participating in a psilocybin clinical trial. The liver is involved in psilocybin metabolism.[133]

Seizure conditions

Epilepsy or non-epileptic seizures are other conditions that prohibit people from participating in most psilocybin clinical trials. That's likely because, although rare, seizures have been reported following psilocybin use.[134]

Mental health conditions

Psilocybin and other psychedelic trips can be emotionally challenging and temporarily destabilizing, even if you have the best of trips. One concern is that psilocybin could exacerbate existing psychotic symptoms, and rare reports do exist of people having suicidal thoughts or engaging in self-harm while under the influence of psilocybin.[135]

For these reasons, most psilocybin clinical trials exclude people who have a mental health disorder or history of one (or even people with an immediate family history of mental health conditions). Conditions include, but are not limited to, major depressive disorder, schizophrenia, psychotic disorders, bipolar disorder, borderline personality disorder, other personality disorders, suicidal ideation or attempts, and drug and alcohol addictions.

Of course, various studies and clinical trials are aimed at assessing psilocybin's effects in people with some of these conditions. After all, psilocybin, although not a miracle cure, shows potential for helping with some mental health issues (as you'll read in Chapter Eleven). But more research is needed.

What do I need to know about psilocybin with medications or other drugs?

As with many things related to psychedelics, we need more research on potential interactions between psilocybin and prescription or over-the-counter medications or other substances. Psilocybin on its own is a mind-altering substance that causes an intense journey, so I don't recommend taking it with other such substances like alcohol, cannabis, or other psychedelics. However, people do sometimes add cannabis somewhere in their journey. Again, I'm not personally making any combo recommendations.

Since psilocybin impacts serotonin transmission, some concern exists over the potential for interaction with prescription medications that also cause changes to serotonin pathways, including many antidepressants, antipsychotics, mood stabilizers, and more.[136]

A systematic review published in 2022 looked at existing literature from clinical trials and epidemiological studies (of which there were few) on psilocybin and drug interactions. However, the research did provide a few insights.[137] Medications that block the 5-HT$_{2A}$ receptor may reduce the effects of psilocybin. These include, but are not limited to, buspirone (a medication to treat anxiety), chlorpromazine and risperidone (both antipsychotics), and ketanserin (used to treat high blood pressure). Medications that are dopamine (D2) receptor antagonists, such as haloperidol (an antipsychotic), seem to exacerbate anxiety or unease when taken with psilocybin. Additionally, research shows that escitalopram, a selective serotonin reuptake inhibitor (SSRI)—used to treat depression and anxiety—that blocks the action of the serotonin transporter, does not lessen psilocybin's effects. However, it does appear to reduce feelings of distress. The researchers theorize that other medications that block the action of the serotonin transporter would have a similar effect.[138]

Most psilocybin clinical trials require participants to taper off antidepressants prior to the study. One concern is serotonin syndrome, a condition that can be life-threatening. However, psilocybin, when combined with a single antidepressant, hasn't been shown to up this risk.[139] Taking multiple medications along with psilocybin may be another story. Ultimately, we need more research to understand all possible medication interactions.

If you're on any medications to treat underlying conditions, don't suddenly stop taking them; always consult your doctor. And if you're on medications for a mental health condition, such as depression, anxiety, a mood disorder, etc., and you want to try psilocybin, I again recommend having a conversation with your doctor or reaching out to another healthcare professional who has robust knowledge about psychedelics. They may suggest a safe tapering schedule or offer another solution.

Will I have a never-ending trip?

One concern with psychedelics, albeit a rare one, is hallucinogenic-persisting perception disorder. HPPD is characterized as visual distortions, hallucinations, and other experiences reminiscent of a psychedelic trip that persist, or intermittently occur, after a trip is over. *The Diagnostic and Statistical Manual of Mental Disorders, Fifth Edition* (DSM-5) lists the prevalence rate of this condition to be 4.5 percent of all hallucinogenic users.[140] An extensive research review of case studies found 97 people presenting with HPPD. The researchers categorized the patients by the drug they ingested. In the hallucinogen group—which included psilocybin—LSD was the drug of choice for more than 78 percent.[141] The symptoms of HPPD have also been linked to alcohol use as well as benzodiazepines, so they're not specific to psychedelics. In addition, the symptoms are associated with the use of cannabis, and they've been noted in the general population.[142]

Can psilocybin cause me to permanently lose my mind?

That's a doozy of a question, but an important one. Myths about psychedelics have abounded for decades. One such myth is the idea that psychedelics can cause psychosis in people who otherwise don't exhibit psychotic behavior. Researchers went to work investigating whether there was a link. In one study, they surveyed more than 130,000 people about their drug use. Of the participants, about 20,000 (14 percent) reported having used either psilocybin, LSD, or mescaline—which are all psychedelics—at least once. The researchers did not find a link between psychedelic use and an increased likelihood of recent psychological distress. Ultimately, they failed to find evidence that psychedelic use is a risk factor on its own for mental health issues.[143]

Should I do a guided experience or DIY?

You have several options to consider when planning for a psilocybin journey, including whether to curate your own experience or seek a guided one. What you choose will depend on your unique situation.

Access to guided experiences is complicated—often because of travel logistics, laws, cost, or a combination of these reasons. Here, I outline the different guided options for trying psilocybin. (If you're planning a DIY trip, Chapter Ten is all about logistics and best practices.)

For guided options, you have several choices, including enrolling in a clinical trial, opting for psilocybin-assisted psychotherapy, going to a psilocybin-specific retreat, or finding an experienced guide to help you with a personalized session. Each of these options has its own considerations pertaining to safety and trip experience.

One consideration that pertains to all situations: Be aware of exactly who will be with you during a trip and, if you're with a guide, shaman, or therapist, find out about their methods or practices first. As noted in the section on psilocybin's effects on the brain, psychedelics have a way of dissolving boundaries between self and other. Plus, psychedelics are mind-altering substances, and they may impart suggestibility.[144] Both factors have major implications for consent and, therefore, sexual assault. (I cover this in Chapter Six.)

Clinical trials

Volunteering for a clinical trial is one way to partake in a guided and supervised psilocybin session, especially if you like the idea of contributing to the growing body of research on psilocybin and psychedelics in general. You can search for a clinical trial on ClinicalTrials.gov. Depending on the clinical trial and its current phase, it may exclude people with certain underlying conditions or who take certain medications. However, some phases of clinical trials will be studying how psilocybin affects or impacts people with a specific underlying condition or who take a specific medication, so you may be able to find a clinical trial that fits your exact situation.

Clinical trials are conducted by a mix of researchers, medical professionals, and staff; that can be a plus if you have concerns related to your physical or mental health. Of course, clinical trials do have some drawbacks. Although psychedelic studies generally take care to incorporate elements of set and setting (discussed in Chapter Ten), they're still—by their nature—clinical, so you likely won't be out in nature enjoying the trees, for example. Plus, you may also have to travel to get to a study location, though you may be compensated for your expenses as well as your time. Additionally, not everyone can get into a clinical trial or get into one exactly when they want to.

If you do seek participation in a clinical trial, find out who will be present with you during your session, what your session will entail, and what to expect immediately after and later with follow-up. Will you receive integration therapy, for example? With whom and for how many sessions? Will you incur any expenses?

Psilocybin-assisted psychotherapy

Psilocybin-assisted psychotherapy, or PAP (I know, not a great acronym!), is exactly what it sounds like. You take psilocybin under the supervision and guidance of a therapist or other facilitator. As of the writing of this book, there isn't a consistent framework for what PAP is from country to country or from state to state in the United States, so I'm just going to go ahead and call it a bit of a Wild West situation when it comes to processes, ethics, and more. Please read Chapter Six if you're considering psychedelic-assisted psychotherapy.

Psychedelic retreats

You can find a host of psilocybin-specific retreats that essentially curate the entire psychedelic experience for you. A benefit of a retreat may include the incorporation of ceremony, which can help get you into the right mindset for your psilocybin journey. Another benefit might be the social aspect. Depending on the structure of the retreat, other people may be embarking on a psychedelic experience with you, which can create a sense of unity and camaraderie. Of course, that can also be a drawback of a retreat. Other than any companions you invite on your adventure, you won't have control over who is around you, and that can raise issues of safety. Additionally, being in a large group may either positively or negatively influence your experience. Remember, psilocybin affects everyone differently each time they go on a journey. If someone you're with is working through a heavy trauma, that may change your trip. That's not to say you shouldn't go on a retreat; it's simply a consideration.

I recommend doing your homework about any retreat you're considering. Find out the facility's safety protocols. How does the retreat handle medical emergencies? Let's say you're highly allergic to bee stings, for example, and you get stung while seriously tripping. Will the facility administer your rescue medications and get you the appropriate professional medical attention? Also find out the retreat's ceremonial processes, how many people will participate, what happens after a psilocybin journey (such as whether therapy is included), etc. Read all the online reviews you can get your eyes on.

Other guided options

If you read the first chapter, you learned about my personalized guided retreat with Gabriel Castillo and Bridgette Rivera at Finally Detached. Castillo is a self-described initiated *curandero* (native healer) and psychedelic guide. I researched extensively to find a way to have a personalized guided retreat, and Finally Detached became my plan A. I'm glad I went with plan A because I couldn't have asked for a better experience. Finally Detached checked all the boxes by incorporating safety, preparation, guidance, ceremony, appropriate emotional support during and after, and follow-up. Yet my guides never interfered with my trip. Instead, they let me experience my psilocybin journey as it unfolded in a safe environment and stood by in case I needed anything. (If you need resource recommendations that might be able to help you find safe guides or other practitioners, see Chapter Six.)

If you enlist the services of a guide or trip sitter whom you don't know, I recommend extensive homework. Depending on your personal circumstances, you may want a female trip sitter or to have both a male and female present, though these aren't fail-safe precautions. You may also wish to have a safety person, such as a sober friend who will join you. Whomever you enlist as a guide, you should have a consultation with this person or people—either a phone or video chat—to get a feel for them. Find out if they have reviews or referrals they can share. Ask them about their process for a guided journey. Make sure you feel a good vibe with them. They should also screen you. They should be asking you about underlying conditions or medications, any history of trauma, any history of suicidal ideation, whether you're dealing with something particularly heavy, your intentions for using psilocybin, etc. Also be mindful of exchanging money. Obviously, you will have to pay for a person's services at some point in the process. Just take care against scams.

Whether you're embarking on a guided journey or more of a DIY route, the logistics info (see Chapter Ten) can help set you up for an optimal trip. Plus, that's where you'll find info about microdosing.

Chapter 6

SEXUAL HEALTH and PSILOCYBIN

Consent concerns, plus psilocybin's sex life-enhancing potential

If you felt like the entire safety chapter was simply a referral to this chapter, there's a huge reason for that. Yes, the research surrounding psilocybin and other psychedelics is exciting. But, at the same time, some nefarious guides, shamans, and therapists have harmed people seeking psychedelic experiences.[145]

This chapter is broken into two main sections: The first part is on consent and boundaries in the context of psilocybin sessions with facilitators, and the second is about the topic of sex life and psilocybin. I've put these two topics together because without consent you've got assault or rape.

I also want to be clear about something: by including content on consent in a psilocybin book for women, I'm not suggesting that only women endure sexual assault. One in six men has been sexually abused or assaulted.[146] And that stat is likely low, considering that men are less likely than women to report or disclose assault. Additionally, research indicates high rates of sexual assault perpetrated against nonbinary people.[147]

What do I need to know about consent, boundaries, and abuses of power?

In the safety chapter, I mentioned *New York* magazine's podcast *Cover Story: Power Trip*, cocreated, produced, and reported by Lily Kay Ross, PhD, and David Nickles, both team members of the nonprofit Psymposia. They've done an excellent job of reporting on the abuses of power occurring in the psychedelics industry, particularly those perpetrated by therapists, guides, and shamans against unsuspecting clients.[148] If you haven't given it a listen, I strongly encourage doing so. Any summarization on my part would be inadequate at best.

Natalie Villeneuve, MSW, RSW, not involved with the podcast, describes the issue with some therapists and guides: "Facilitators have breached boundaries or have had sexual relations with their participants," she says. "And the participant in that moment and afterwards feels like it was okay because they were convinced that it was okay under the influence or it felt really good in a lot of ways during the time." It's sometimes not until later, if at all, that the client names it for what it was: abuse. "There's no circumstance," Villeneuve says, "where someone who is in a position of power over you while you're under the influence of a psychedelic medication—that they should be having any kind of sexual relationship with you."

I came across Villeneuve's work at Psychedemia, a conference on psychedelics, where she presented a poster on "Sexual Abuse and Ethical Misconduct in Psychedelic Therapies: Ways Forward in the Wake of Controversies." She's written about the topic, and her work in this area is ongoing. "The hope is to establish something that provides this safety network for people that makes it easier for them," she explains in our phone interview. "Right now, that's not in place. There's no system of oversight for people who are practicing psychedelic therapy. There's no way to navigate whether people have caused harm or not." The system she describes will take time to build, but she provides insight on how people seeking psychedelic-assisted therapy—or guided experiences in general—can vet practitioners in the meantime.

Vulnerability and suggestibility

"Since I've started getting into this work," Villeneuve says, "I've also been really torn because I still have a positive view of psychedelics and think that they have enormous potential and personally appreciate the benefits of them." But at the same time, she expresses worry. "I always get a knot in my stomach when someone's like, 'Oh, I'm doing this thing. I'm doing an ayahuasca experience ...' I get really nervous about that because of what's been going on." She's referring to abuses of power by guides, shamans, and therapists. "People who are [seeking] these therapies," she says, "may have their own histories of trauma. And when you have a history of trauma, you don't have the best gauge on relationships and what's safe or what's not."

Some practitioners seem to be taking advantage of that vulnerable state of their clients. Then consider that psilocybin and other psychedelics, by their actions on the brain, can make us even more vulnerable. Remember, you can feel incredibly open or connected to others.[149] A psychedelic experience can also increase one's suggestibility.[150] For example, even if you're opposed to any form of touch during your psychedelic journey, someone may be able to convince you it's what you need or want in the moment.

I think about what doctoral researcher Abigail Calder, MSc, points out in her email answers to my questions on neuroplasticity (a topic discussed in Chapter Three). She shares the details of what her colleague Gregor Hasler, MD, calls the "helioscope effect."[151] A quick refresh: It's the idea that psychedelics can bring up painful or traumatic memories and let you view and even process them without them becoming overwhelming. However, Calder cautions that a therapist who pushes their patient and doesn't let this phenomenon unfold naturally can undermine the effect.

After thinking about this, it's my opinion that an irresponsible or ill-intending guide or therapist could push when their client is most vulnerable, making them even more vulnerable.

Touch

Villeneuve and I have a long conversation about consent and its intersection with psychedelics. I ask her if touch should ever even be a part of psychedelic-assisted therapy, since I'm unsure whether touch is ever appropriate in therapy in general. Touch might be a part of regular therapy (meaning where psychedelics aren't used) in some circumstances, she tells me. "Touch is a normal part of the human experience," Villeneuve explains. "And part of what you're doing in therapy is trying to establish, or reestablish, what safe relationships look like or get people to become grounded in healthy relationships or connection."

But she expresses this with caution—especially when considering the stories coming out in *Cover Story: Power Trip* and elsewhere— about abuses of power in psychedelic-assisted therapy. "That's what therapists are doing now who are causing harm," she says. "They're using that argument of 'Oh, it was for the client's benefit, and this is why.'" But, as she points out, "A hug—it's not going to be life changing." If a hug doesn't occur, it's not going to be the thing preventing someone from healing. A coerced and nonconsensual hug is another story. "If it does happen, it can lead to a lot of harm," Villeneuve adds.

In the context of psychedelic-assisted therapy, touch can be even murkier. "If you've had your boundaries violated," Villeneuve says, "you may not understand what's an appropriate boundary. And when you are really putting your trust into your facilitator to be caring and supportive, you would be counting on them to keep you safe."

You have the right to say no to any type of touch, whether on a retreat, in a therapist's treatment room, with a psychedelic guide, or wherever—end of story. Or you may be thinking therapeutic touch, like a hug, might be something you'd value as part of your journey. Either way, here are some considerations for navigating the concept of touch in a psychedelic setting.

"It needs to be a conversation that's had before being under the influence of anything," Villeneuve says. A thorough conversation sets clear boundaries while you're sober. That way, while you're under the influence, she adds, "you can't say yes to anything you didn't previously consent to, but you can say no." For example, if you agreed well before ingesting psilocybin that holding your hand during the session would be okay but you no longer want that touch in the session, you can revoke that consent at any time. But if while sober, you did not agree to a hug, you can't then say under the influence of psilocybin that a hug is okay. "That's not true consent," Villeneuve explains. The responsibility is on your guide or therapist to honor the consent conversation and boundaries you set while you were sober. And they shouldn't pressure you into any form of touch—ever.

FRIES

To further examine this topic, Villeneuve walks me through the acronym she uses to explain consent to the teens she works with. To be clear, she does not work with teens in a psychedelic context, but for the sake of our conversation, she ties her examples to psychedelic settings. The acronym is FRIES. "Consent is freely given. It's reversible. It's informed. It's enthusiastic. And it's specific," she explains.

Freely given means you're not under the influence and you're not being coerced or manipulated into giving it. In the context of a psilocybin session, you might have a pre-session conversation like the one just described about touch. Your practitioner might offer an example of how touch, like holding your hand, may be helpful during a session. But if you say no and they push it, that's persuasion. "That's not consensual," Villeneuve says.

Reversible means you always have the right to change your mind about anything you've consented to so far, no matter where you are in the session. But the reversal only works one way: A *yes* can always become a *no*. But if you've said no to something pre-session, you can't change your *no* to a *yes* during the session.

"*Informed* means you know exactly what you're getting into when you say yes to it," Villeneuve explains. A guide or therapist should be clear with you beforehand about exactly what to expect during a session.

Enthusiastic in the context of a sexual experience (not related to psychedelics) means, as Villeneuve puts it, "you're super into it, you're agreeing to it, you're not just like, 'Oh yeah, maybe.'" She adds, "I always say consent is not about waiting for someone to stop." When it comes to a psychedelic-assisted therapy session, sex should never be part of the equation. The point is that a therapist or guide has a role in understanding your body language as well as what you're telling them. "In a psilocybin experience," Villeneuve says, "if someone's just like, 'I'm not sure if that would be right for me,' that's not enthusiastic."

Specific, Villeneuve says, means that consent is required for everything before it occurs. "In the context of psilocybin therapy," she explains, "each piece of what you're doing is spoken about beforehand. The *informed* and *specific* pieces really tie together here. You know exactly what you're getting into and there's consent for each individual thing along the way." An example might be that you're aware ahead of time and have consented to the idea that the therapist might hold your hand. But in the session, if they are then thinking of holding your hand as a form of comfort, they should still ask and ensure you've given consent before doing so.

Red flags

We both want to be clear about something before launching into this topic. "It's never on the person to prevent sexual abuse," Villeneuve says. "But there are, I think, red flags you can look out for."

Search their name. See if anything comes up regarding allegations of abuse or other questionable practices.

Ask questions. Find out about the guide's or therapist's background, training, and values and whether they receive guidance for the work they do. "Do they receive clinical supervision?" Villeneuve asks regarding therapists. One thing that's a common practice in psychedelic-assisted therapy is having two therapists, usually one male and one female, in the room. "We don't have enough knowledge or information right now to establish whether or not that's the standard protocol," Villeneuve says. As we've learned from the accounts shared in *Cover Story: Power Trip*, that practice hasn't prevented all harm. Villeneuve shares a personal concern—one I agree with. "I find it really concerning when husbands and wives do this together or people who are partnered," she says. "Why I say husbands and wives specifically is because there are husbands and wives who have been doing this work and who have abused people." She's careful to point out that of course therapists in partnered relationships have done great work together, so she's not implying that such work as a whole is problematic. But she makes a good point. "What kind of power dynamic does that create," she says, "when you're with the person you're married to and you're providing therapy to someone that's extremely intimate and where they're very vulnerable?" The issue is that the couple already has an intimate relationship involving love and sexuality. Then they're working to help someone else who is looking to them for guidance. "It just creates a dynamic," Villeneuve adds, "that, to me, amplified by a psychedelic medicine, is just so concerning."

Have a meeting (or several) where psychedelics aren't part of the equation. This won't be an option for all scenarios. But in the case of psychedelic-assisted therapy, you may be able to have a session that's psilocybin free first to get a feel for someone. "I always tell people in the context of regular therapy," Villeneuve says, "it takes time to find the right therapist for you." You may be able to consult with a guide beforehand, whether in person or virtually, as well. For me, that option was a sign that my guide had my best interests in mind.

Trust your gut. Maybe you're traveling to Mexico for a psychedelic retreat, Villeneuve offers as an example. But then, on the first day, something feels off because the retreat is not what you expected or a facilitator makes a comment to you that doesn't feel right. Know that you can leave. "We often ignore these gut feelings or these red flags," she says.

Talk to others. They can "help you establish whether or not your gut feeling is just some nerves or if it's actually something like one of these red flags," Villeneuve explains.

Have a plan B. If you do go on a retreat or otherwise travel for a psychedelic experience, have a plan for getting out of the situation if you need to. That might mean having the option to change your flight or having backup lodging, Villeneuve suggests.

Resources

Communities of like-minded psilocybin and other psychedelic users—or those interested in trying psychedelics—are growing. They can serve as a resource to you when seeking safe guides or therapists, asking questions, or bouncing ideas.

One such community is Sisters in Psychedelics.[152] SIP is a community of female-identifying people who are passionate about safe and intentional psychedelic use. SIP, founded by Bea Chan and Dana Harvey, in Vancouver, British Columbia, was originally born out of a potluck hangout in November 2021. It has since grown into an international community. SIP features a free online platform, as well as online and in-person events, including the annual SIP Summit. "It is always about elevating the voices of women, the divine feminine, and other underrepresented voices," Chan explains in our phone conversation.

I ask Chan about the potential for abuses of power in the psychedelic space. "I'm really sad to say that this is real," Chan says. "It's happened. It's been in the news. I personally know somebody who has been assaulted in a medicine ceremony before. And it's just really sad to have to acknowledge this is real." She echoes Villeneuve's advice on researching anyone you'll be working with. "Really do your homework," Chan says, "on who is trip sitting you, who is your therapist, who is going to be your guide."

SIP's online platform is a place where you can talk to other SIP members and engage in community and connection. "We are all for referring our own trusted therapist or underground sitter or things like that," Chan says.

Another resource is Psychedelic Survivors.[153] This website and online community supports survivors of abuse, assault, and personal harm that occurred in a psychedelic setting or context. The organizers are Leia Friedwoman, MS, and Katherine MacLean, PhD. They are working on a project called "Psychedelic Safety Flags," which they say is "a color system to assess underground practitioner ethics and safety." As of the writing of this book, the project isn't live online yet, but once I have a link to it, I will post it on my socials. Psychedelic Safety Flags uses a color system to note different degrees of power dynamics, consent, and more. As you might guess, a red flag would denote facilitators who disregard boundaries and consent. A green one would indicate facilitators who discuss boundaries and honor them.

Can magic mushrooms add magic to my sex life?

Again, I'm including the topic of sex in the same chapter regarding consent because you can't have one without the other—or it's called rape or assault. I'm *mostly* approaching the sex-life topic from the lens of sex while not tripping on magic mushrooms, though I cover some aspects of that as well in this section. Shrooms might be a sex-life-enhancing tool because of their potential for boosting mood, spurring personal growth, forging connection, and more (all things discussed in Chapter Three).

First, let's explore the topic of women's sexual health and pleasure and the disparities in care for female sexual dysfunction. Roughly 40 percent of women of reproductive age endure some type of sexual dysfunction, whether that's with libido, the enjoyment of sex, or reaching orgasm.[154] And for those who've surpassed the menopause milestone, 85 percent experience sexual dysfunction.[155] The World Health Organization says, "Sexual health is fundamental to the overall health and well-being of individuals, couples and families, and to the social and economic development of communities and countries."[156] A hallmark of female sexual dysfunction is personal distress, which contributes to reduced quality of life.[157]

At the same time, barriers exist for people assigned female at birth to receive treatment for sexual dysfunction, and many barriers involve gaps in our healthcare system. These include a lack of healthcare-provider education and training on the topic and the individual biases they bring to the exam table. Sexual medicine objectives aren't widely included in residency programs.[158] Plus, medicine didn't even have a complete understanding of clitoral anatomy until 2005, when Helen O'Connell, MD, a urologist, and her colleagues used functional magnetic resonance imaging (fMRI) to map out, for the first time, the full clitoris, including its internal structures.[159] The penis, however, has received much more research attention. The FDA approved the first medication for erectile dysfunction, one of the most common male sexual concerns, in 1998.[160] The most common form of sexual dysfunction for women is hypoactive sexual desire disorder (HSDD), basically a severe lack of sex drive. The FDA approved the first medication for female HSDD nearly 17 years later in 2015.[161] So to recap, a drug for male sexual dysfunction existed seven years before the medical establishment even had a complete concept of the clitoris. Then it took an entire decade before a drug for female sexual dysfunction hit the market. Clearly, women's sexual health and pleasure have not been a priority in the medical field. These disparities in care lead to stigma.

Research on psilocybin is still ongoing in many areas. So far, I haven't found research directly linking magic mushroom use to enhanced sex life for people assigned female at birth. But I think there's potential in this area. Many factors—including physical, psychological, and social—can contribute to female sexual dysfunction. And in no way would I want to present shrooms as some sort of sexual-health panacea. I hope research ensues in a safe and productive way.

In the meantime, I think there are some things to consider. Low libido is linked to depression.[162] And we know that psilocybin has mood-elevating potential, so it's not a stretch to hypothesize that a mood boost might potentiate a bedroom boost. Factors that can contribute to sexual dysfunction include sexual abuse or rape.[163] A history of sexual and emotional abuse is associated with vaginismus, which is the involuntary tensing or contraction of vaginal muscles upon penetration. And a history of sexual abuse is associated with dyspareunia—painful intercourse.[164] A meta-analysis of more than 2,000 survivors of sexual assault found that nearly 75 percent met the criteria for a PTSD diagnosis within the first month after the assault.[165] More research is needed regarding psilocybin's potential to help with trauma.[166] But early clinical trials on psilocybin and PTSD are in the works.[167] (See Chapter Eleven.) Research shows that factors that help protect against sexual dysfunction include intimate communication and having a positive body image.[168] And experts suggest psilocybin may be able to help in those areas.

For expertise, I reach out to Michele Ross, PhD. She's a neuroscientist who wrote an article about sex and shrooms.[169] Psilocybin can aid with self-discovery, which can then lead to new discoveries when you're partnered up. "I always think that solo work and solo trips are really important," Ross explains, "because when you are in touch with yourself and you're more confident, when you go into the bedroom, you bring that confidence. You're more able to voice what you need with your partner, you're more able to connect—bring your authentic self."

Ross shares her story of a 2-gram private psilocybin self-love journey. "I went dancing in the moonlight and got a little horny out there and masturbated," she says. "You've got to love yourself, love your curves, love how your body's changing—love all your parts." She embarked on her adventure during the last full moon, reflecting on having turned 40.

Whether you're tripping with another person or solo, you may feel an enhanced sense of connection in the moment or post-trip to the people you love, and that, too, may have benefits in the bedroom. "When you're more connected to your partner," Ross says, "obviously sex can be better—when you're more attentive to each other's needs. It really depends on what you think better sex is." That could mean more orgasms, longer orgasms, more variety in positions—the list goes on. Better sex may involve keeping things interesting. "I think seeing couples that are especially older," Ross adds, "discovering magic mushrooms and incorporating that into their relationship, I think that's really interesting."

Ross addresses some of the issues that may occur when considering sex life and psilocybin, especially when the two are mixed. "Psilocybin can sort of make you connect but make you not want to have sex," she says. It's also important to realize that a mushroom trip isn't always light and fun. "Wounds and trauma can be brought up," Ross explains. In other words, psilocybin isn't a classic aphrodisiac.

Of course, the topic of consent comes into play, as well. If you are merging psilocybin and sex, Ross says to set boundaries before ingesting substances. "It really is important that if somebody wants to stop at any point," she explains, "somebody should be allowed to stop and leave the experience."

Drugs, including alcohol, can obviously impair or incapacitate someone from consenting.[170] So I ask Villeneuve about sex while on psychedelics between two enthusiastic, consenting adults. "Outside of psilocybin," she says, "this is where people get kind of tripped up sometimes in terms of consent." She's referring to the concept that you must be completely sober to consent. "Well, think of how many drunk people have sex all of the time, right?" she says. "It's not about like, 'Oh, now that's rape because you are drunk and you had sex.' No. It's about what does that level of influence do to your ability to kind of understand the situation or consent to certain things." Using the FRIES acronym, two consenting adults, especially ones who know each other well intimately, can continue to navigate consent while somewhat under the influence.

The next chapter provides a peek at how one woman and her husband have used psilocybin to foster connection and improve their relationship.

Chapter 7

EMMA'S STORY

**An improved relationship
and relief from anxiety**

Emma reaches out to me on social media after I announce I am writing this book. She expresses excitement regarding the content and tells me she and her husband have had some transformative experiences on psychedelics, including psilocybin. I ask if I can interview her. For various reasons, she asks me not to share her real name, so Emma is a pseudonym.

A diagnosis of anxiety

Emma, now in her early forties, grew up in the "just say no" era, which was rife with falsehoods like, as she puts it, "They're drugs. If you try that one time, your face will melt." But when she met her now husband, he'd had an array of experience with not only cannabis but also psychedelics—and he was doing just fine.

By that time, Emma had been struggling with anxiety for nearly a decade. The anxiety cropped up after college when she faced uncertainty about what the rest of her life would look like. Emma would ruminate to the point of getting an upset stomach, she recalls. Her doctor sent her to a psychologist, who then gave her a prescription for an SSRI. The medication worked well for several years, but then Emma went to grad school and things changed. "I kind of just felt my anxiety spiraling out of control," she says. Her doctor upped her dosage. "But there were some side effects to that," Emma adds. Over time, she found that tools like cognitive behavioral therapy and a small amount of cannabis often helped her anxiety—both without those same side effects as her SSRI. With the help of her doctor, she tapered off the prescription.

Additionally, knowing how psilocybin had benefited her partner, she was curious how magic mushrooms might help her—especially since, with him, she had a safe person and environment for experimenting. On a sunny Saturday afternoon, in her partner's apartment, the two ingested a small dose of the Golden Teacher strain. "He said, 'We're just going to hang out and watch *SpongeBob* and see how you feel,'" she recalls. "I did feel something. Colors were kind of brighter, and I just had a really lightweight, fun feeling."

From there, Emma started to take deeper, longer trips, some of which have been darker. "The way I look at it," she says, "is that you don't get the trip you want; you get the trip you need, and it might not be what you were exactly prepared to deal with at the time. But you're going to get through it." Her advice: "Don't try to fight it."

Those challenging trips—or just parts of trips—have netted growth. On a particularly difficult journey, one in which she says she turned to her husband and asked, "Did we die?" she later had an insight about herself. At one point, she started getting flashes of every friendship she'd ever had. "It was like they were just backed up and laid out," she recalls, "in a way that kind of let me look at them all at the same time and be like, 'Oh, why do I always do that?' And it was something about holding myself back so I would be accepted."

Intense and uncomfortable trip experiences have encouraged her to confront her anxiety. "I was able to separate," she says, "and be like, 'Ha, look! Look at that thing. You don't have to do that to yourself. It doesn't have to be this way. Here's an alternate way.'" Viewing her anxiety responses and facing them head-on during a trip, she adds, allowed her to identify them later when not tripping and change the trajectory. Now she says she's better equipped to ease or stop anxiety in everyday experiences. "Psilocybin in particular," she explains, "it's a facilitator of both you getting in touch with your own emotions but also you being able to process that after the fact and try to incorporate that more into your life."

Opening communication lines

Meaningful trips have spurred growth in her marriage, as well. "It's absolutely deepened our relationship," Emma says. "It's made us able to talk about things that are hard and acknowledge things about ourselves that are hard but also can be changed." She describes a trip in which she and her husband both experienced what she calls a "paradigm shift," where everything—meaning the whole universe—was going to be okay. It's a sensation she's been able to return to in subsequent trips, but it also helped Emma and her husband make strides together. Emma says they used to have the usual minor squabbles that occur when two people are starting to merge their lives and trying to get on the same page. After their paradigm-shift trip, however, they both continued to feel the undercurrent that everything would somehow be okay. "I think we were just a little gentler with each other after that point," she says. "You know, let's do better by each other." She describes psilocybin as a catalyst for improved communication, which helps each of them to understand where the other one is coming from.

Although she hasn't reached for psilocybin in about two years, she and her husband used to turn to magic mushrooms for what she refers to as a "mental reset" a few times a year. "There's a little bit of a glow the next day," she says. "[I] just feel lighter and happier, and it tends to last."

Chapter 8

PARENTING and PSILOCYBIN

Pregnancy, breastfeeding/ chestfeeding, and family life with psilocybin

At first consideration, it may seem like there isn't a whole lot to say about pregnancy and breastfeeding/chestfeeding and psilocybin—other than the snippet I included in the Q&A section. But there *is* so much more to say. Plus, we've also got the topic of parenting and psilocybin to consider. So parenting as a whole—whether you're a birthing parent, someone who is breastfeeding/chestfeeding, or someone who has kids of any age—gets its own chapter.

When I start investigating these topics, I am not surprised to see there's a dearth of information and research out there. Yet we've got plenty of questions. What are the safety considerations for psilocybin while pregnant or nursing? What about if a birthing parent needs care for their mental health? And what are the considerations, stigmas, concerns, barriers, and potential benefits for parents when it comes to using psilocybin? Even after researching, I don't have definitive answers for you, but I at least have nuanced information from some key experts and parents.

What's the info on psilocybin use while pregnant or breastfeeding/chestfeeding?

Basically, zero research exists on using psilocybin while pregnant. I shouldn't say zero, since some studies of pregnant rats do exist. But you're not a rat! Pregnant people are automatically excluded from psychedelic clinical trials. Rather than an abundance of data, we're dealing with an absence of information on how psilocybin affects a fetus.

"The challenge with doing any peer-reviewed, evidence-based research in pregnancy is that it's not ethical," Rebecca Kronman, LCSW, tells me in our phone interview. "We're not asking a pregnant person to ingest a particular substance and then see what it does to the developing fetus." We also don't have clinical trials on the effects of psilocybin in human milk. But the topic of psychedelics and pregnancy or breastfeeding/chestfeeding is more nuanced than that.

In her private practice, Kronman helps patients prepare for psychedelic experiences and to integrate after. She's also the founder of Plant Parenthood,[171] which is a virtual and in-person community of "parents but also nonparents who are looking at the intersection of psychedelics in the family system," she explains. "The mission of the organization is to destigmatize this topic and bring difficult conversations forward."

Kronman wrote an in-depth article about the topic of psychedelics and pregnancy for *Psychedelics Today*.[172] With the absence of data, blanket statements regarding substance use while pregnant or breastfeeding/chestfeeding exist. Kronman outlines some of them in her comprehensive article.[173] For example, the American College of Obstetricians and Gynecologists recommends avoiding marijuana use.[174] ACOG lumps psilocybin and other psychedelics into a category noted as "substances that are commonly misused or abused."[175] That categorization is rooted in myth and clearly hasn't kept up with research on psilocybin's therapeutic potential. A blanket statement surrounding psychedelic use while pregnant or breastfeeding/chestfeeding leaves out a lot of context.

"When we're trying to get answers to our concerns about what is safe to ingest," Kronman says, "we really have to think about using other spaces of knowledge." Kronman explains that—outside the Western medicine research model—we can consider how pregnant or nursing people or parents in other cultures approach psilocybin." That's just one example.

I also interview Hilary Agro, an anthropologist and PhD candidate at the University of British Columbia. "There are groups of Indigenous people who intentionally use mushrooms while they're breastfeeding," she says. "I have done all this research on pregnancy and breastfeeding and drugs. And there is no evidence that psychedelics or especially psilocybin has a negative effect. It doesn't mean you should do it all the time."

Kronman adds, "We want to be careful not to be too reductionist about this and say, 'Well those kids are doing fine.'"

To summarize the info on safety, we don't have evidence of harm on a fetus or a nursing child, nor do we have evidence of absolute safety. We need more nuance and open discussions about the topic, and these discussions warrant robust consideration in the broader scope of health and well-being for the pregnant or nursing person. "Gestating parents deserve bodily autonomy too," Agro says. "You don't just become a carrier who has to sacrifice everything for your baby."

Agro is vocal in her public-facing educational work about her experience with attention deficit hyperactivity disorder (ADHD). She's been pregnant twice. "I tried to go off of my ADHD meds, and it did not work," she says. "And it was bad for me. And it was going to be worse for the pregnancy to be unmedicated because I can't eat properly. It was going to be worse for my babies to be off of my medication, but importantly it was going to be worse for me."

The number of pregnant people taking ADHD medication is increasing. And while some research indicates an association with taking ADHD meds during pregnancy with an increased risk of birth defects, that associated risk is quite low.[176] The research to date on the topic is limited and based on small numbers of children, so more research is needed. I share the ADHD research here only to illustrate that, yeah, research is limited on all sorts of drugs, not just psilocybin, regarding pregnancy and breastfeeding/chestfeeding. Ultimately, birthing and lactating parents must make the best choices for themselves and their families—as Agro has done—with the help of any trusted experts in their corner.

"We have to question the use of substances for purely recreational purposes during this period," Kronman says, "but if we're talking about things that are really keeping the birthing parent alive—and we know that there are psychedelics that truly are imparting that function—then we would really need to consider and weigh out against the unknown risk."

The health of the birthing parent is paramount. Plus, the birthing or nursing parent's health also impacts the health of a developing fetus or their already-born child. "We know that things like depression, PTSD, and anxiety can negatively impact someone's ability to attach to their baby," Kronman explains. These mental health concerns, both during pregnancy and after birth, can also affect child development.[177] Adequate and compassionate treatment is crucial.

"These are not definitive answers," Kronman says, "but when we use a harm-reduction approach, we can say, 'Well, what does that risk feel like to me, knowing all the risks or potential risks or unknowns? How do I feel about that practice given the information that I do have on hand?'"

I speak to Mikaela de la Myco, who focuses on womb-healing facilitation in the Ma'at tradition. You can find a course called "Psychedelics & Maternity" that she teaches (in conjunction with other facilitators) via DoubleBlind magazine.[178] I share more from de la Myco in Chapter Eleven, but her pregnancy story belongs here.

"The microdosing experiences that I had as a pregnant person were basically to address the ongoing alcoholism that I was involved in in my life," she says. "The way that I treated microdosing during my pregnancy was as an alternative to drinking." Since age 13, de la Myco had struggled with alcohol. Having been raised by parents with alcohol use disorder, de la Myco wanted something different for her family. "That was a piece of generational trauma that I wanted to address," she says. "The mushrooms, in place of alcohol, gave me the healing key—which I then needed to carry with me—

and eventually changed my life." Psilocybin was a catalyst for a behavioral change that, as she puts it, cleared her relationship with alcohol. (You can find info regarding psilocybin's potential to help with alcohol use disorder in Chapter Eleven.)

"If it's between a pregnant person choosing to use psilocybin three times while they're pregnant," Agro says hypothetically, "and the alternative is they're going to use alcohol 50 times while they're pregnant, there's just a clear better choice there if you take a harm-reduction approach."

I ask Kronman about the topic of psilocybin use while breastfeeding/chestfeeding. She suggests I contact her lactation consultant. Andrea Syms-Brown, IBCLC, immediately agrees to an interview. "We have to understand where this person is coming from," she says, speaking generally—not about a specific parent. "Having compassion for this individual is key to understanding why this use is necessary." Syms-Brown points out that if a lactating parent is turning to psilocybin or another psychedelic, they're likely not doing so for recreational purposes but rather for an aspect related to their health. "Knowing when to use it," she adds, "is usually under the care of a shaman or even a physician who says, 'Okay, this is how we're going to treat this particular illness that you're experiencing.'"

The strategy of psilocybin ingestion and timing of feedings will vary per each family's unique situation. "There's no one rule," Syms-Brown says. "We ask mothers to abstain from breastfeeding at certain times if they're on certain medications because we know when it's highest in the blood. So if we treat these products in the same manner, we can have the same or similar results." With microdosing a single dried dose, you can control the timing easier than you can with, say, sipping a larger dose in several cups of tea, Syms-Brown notes. Not just the dosage, but the age of the child is also a variable, since a newborn will need to feed more often.

Half-life is the time needed for a drug to reduce to half its original dose in the body. The half-life of psilocybin (and psilocin) is roughly three hours.[179] So your dose will have been reduced by 50 percent at this time. You can see why Syms-Brown brings up dosage. A microdose of 0.10 grams of psilocybin would be reduced to about 0.05 grams at around three hours, whereas a 3-gram dose would only be reduced to 1.5 grams at three hours. After 3.3 half-lives of a drug, 90 percent is eliminated.[180] And after 5 half-lives, 98 percent of it should be out of your system, according to the Infant Risk Center.[181] With psilocybin, you'll reach the 3.3 half-life point at about 10 hours and 5 half-lives at 15 hours. Plus, we know that reports show that psilocybin and psilocin are almost completely excreted from urine after 24 hours.[182] This info can help you decide the best strategies for you and your family.

A lactation consultant can also help offer guidance surrounding breastfeeding/chestfeeding and any medication or other substance use. Syms-Brown makes it clear that the role of the lactation consultant does not involve criticism or passing judgment. "Our job is to support breastfeeding and support the families who choose to breastfeed their children," she says. "That's it. So whatever it takes to support that process is what we do. I'm going to give you all the facts and help you to navigate whatever habits you might have so that you can be confident that your baby's getting the best of you."

How do I navigate the intersection of parenting and psilocybin?

We don't have definitive answers or definitive research on some of these topics surrounding parenting and psilocybin—especially those regarding pregnancy or breastfeeding. But having conversations about them helps open lines of communication, reduces stigma, and helps people navigate the psychedelic landscape with care and consideration. "We feel like this is the number one key to safer substance use," says Kronman of Plant Parenthood, "that people are talking about what they're doing—that they're not hiding in the shadows."

Kronman acknowledges that having open conversations surrounding drug use can be complicated. "All of us are steeped in the war on drugs," she says. "It's still well and alive. People are still experiencing consequences from it—in particular, Black and Brown people." In addition, stigma surrounding drug use exists for parents, especially for pregnant people. "The world has eyes on you as a birthing parent and also as a parent with a young child," Kronman notes.

Agro openly identifies as a drug user online and elsewhere. It's her provocative approach to her advocacy work for harm reduction, stigma reduction, and decriminalization, and for people to have bodily autonomy. "We have this common conception of who is a drug user," she says. "There are drug users, which are people who use drugs, and there are regular people. And that is completely inaccurate."

Agro identifies as a drug user for the stimulant medications she takes for ADHD. "I would argue most people on the planet are drug users," she says. Before you say you're not, ask yourself if you drink coffee or other products with caffeine, consume alcohol, or take prescription or over-the-counter medications. That's Agro's point. If you answered yes, you're a drug user. Hey, I'm a drug user. "It's this sort of coming-out-of-the-closet thing," Agro says, "where if we realize, 'Oh, I'm a drug user, you're a drug user, we all are, then why do only some of us go to prison for it?'" The answer is not that some drugs are illegal because they're dangerous. "You can debunk that easily," Agro explains, "because alcohol is legal and it's not the safest drug." Categorizing people as drug users and pitting them against medication takers only perpetuates stigma and harm.

Agro has firsthand experience with that stigma and harm. Shortly after she gave birth in 2021, when she was still recovering from her cesarean section, someone reported her to child protective services, saying that she's a drug abuser and that they fear for her children. Agro wrote a Twitter thread about her experience.[183] A social worker—a kind one, Agro notes—came to her house and inspected her child's body, grilled Agro about her medical history, and more. "The whole thing was very traumatizing," she recalls. "Parents, but especially women, are extra vulnerable to the war on drugs because we get our kids weaponized against us." The situation stressed Agro so much that it impacted her ability to heal from her C-section. Research shows that stress can dramatically slow wound healing at varying rates.[184] Agro says the delayed healing then impacted her ability to parent. And therein lies the irony: someone reported her, calling into question her parenting abilities, and by doing so, they harmed her parenting abilities.

Agro's experience is a key example of why many women, especially those who have kids, are keeping in the dark the medication they need—whether that be cannabis, psilocybin, or birth control pills. Stigma exists. I share her story not to frighten anyone, but to highlight the importance of reducing that stigma. Agro is quick to point out that structural privileges—such as being an academic and having friends who are social workers and lawyers whom she could lean on for guidance—helped her resolve the child protective services case against her. "I encourage people who can," Agro says, "if they are safe to do so—and they are not at risk of state violence the way that many people who use drugs are—I encourage people to identify as a drug user."

Safe circles, such as Plant Parenthood, can help you get the conversation going and empower you to take that further when and if you're ready. "When we can begin to share these things in groups that we feel will understand," Kronman says, "and when that information is held in a safe container, when this conversation is being facilitated in a way where participants can feel safe, then we can start actually having a conversation about what's going on."

What Kronman is gleaning through some of her conversations with other parents who use psychedelics is that they can be a tool in one's parenting arsenal. "We talk to parents all the time," she says, "who say, 'I use these substances not in spite of the fact that I had children or not to get to escape from the fact that I had children, but in order to heal a familial trauma, in order to be more present for my child, in order to show myself the compassion that I needed so that I could pass that along to my child.'"

Through previous research unrelated to this book, I've read a lot about adverse childhood experiences, also called ACEs. ACEs are when a child is exposed to trauma, such as domestic violence, child abuse, the incarceration of a parent, or having a parent with mental illness, just to list a few.[185] Of course, children with ACEs grow up to be adults—and sometimes parents themselves. One in six adults has experienced four or more ACEs. Research looking at more than 2,000 families found that the children of parents with four or more ACEs had a more than threefold risk of experiencing four or more ACEs as well, when compared to kids of parents without ACEs.[186] The researchers note that addressing parental stress may interrupt the cycle of trauma, something that's crucial for kids' health. ACEs can cause both physical and mental health issues for children later in life. Plus, half of the 10 leading causes of death are linked to ACEs.[187] Preventing ACEs has the potential to reduce, by as much as 44 percent, the number of adults who experience depression. Working through one's own traumas can have a huge impact on the health and well-being of one's child. And we know through preliminary research that magic mushrooms, when used therapeutically, may have the potential to help.[188] (See Agro's story of healing trauma via psilocybin in Chapter Nine.)

"Women—we make most of the household decisions," says Bea Chan, of Sisters in Psychedelics.[189] "I do think that we are the glue of the family." She points out the importance of women's mental health for this reason. "What we're teaching to our next generation," Chan says, "and even further from that—there's just so much more impact we can make if we're whole."

In some instances, parents may be using psychedelics themselves to better connect with their kids. "Especially young children, their brains are very entropic," Kronman explains, "which is exactly the effect we're going for when we take psychedelics. So we take psychedelics and then we hang out with our kids. And all of a sudden we can inhabit their world better." Kronman shares the example of engaging in imaginative play. But psilocybin can also boost empathy.[190] "We can resonate with their experience," she notes.

I'm not a parent myself, so I'm wondering if parents in the psychedelic community have unwritten rules surrounding psilocybin use and parenting. My quick and obvious disclaimer: If someone is serving as a sole caregiver for a young child—meaning another caregiver isn't present—they shouldn't be impaired to the point that they're incapacitated from protecting and caring for that child or in a way that otherwise puts that child at risk. So that's the big rule.

Other considerations come into play, however. Kronman notes that in some cases a parent may want to carve out time to have a psychedelic experience as their form of self-care; they may prefer to be temporarily free from other responsibilities. "In that case," she explains, "they maybe wouldn't want their child to be around. And then we hear from other parents who feel like, 'These are practices that benefit me. I want to share this information with my child. I'm going to let them know what I'm doing.'"

A decision to share such information would likely depend on the child's age and if they may benefit from open, intentional, fact-based conversations surrounding the use of mind-altering substances. Such open dialogue in families can be valuable. "I'm going to come at this from a cultural BIPOC lens," says Chan, who is Chinese. "In the Asian community, it's a huge no-no ... this is not something that I can even really openly talk to my parents about." Stigma, though, can lead to harm if, say, an adolescent has questions about psychedelics or other drugs but they can't talk about it with someone they trust who can give them adequate safety info. "Let's have open conversations about this," Chan says, "without fear or shame or guilt."

Kronman notes another consideration when it comes to the intersection of parenting and psychedelic use. "If you are, for example, in a custody battle," she says, "you may not be able to disclose this stuff to your kids without repercussion." Ultimately, there isn't one set of rules or answers that fits every family when it comes to the intersection of psychedelic use and parenting. However, you've got resources and community to lean on. In addition to Plant Parenthood, you can find support via Moms on Mushrooms (M.O.M), founded by Tracey Tee.[191]

Also, lean on yourself as a guide when it comes to psychedelics in general and their intersection with your role as a parent. "These medicines are unique in that they are decidedly non-Western despite the fast flow of pharma coming at them," Kronman says. "But they're not Western medicine, and they shouldn't be used as such. Part of that means checking in with one's own intuition about what you need, how much you need, whether you need it."

Chapter 9

HILARY'S STORY

Processing ADHD trauma

If you just read the parenting chapter, you'll recognize the name Hilary Agro, an anthropologist and PhD candidate at the University of British Columbia. I want to share more about her personal psilocybin story, particularly concerning attention deficit hyperactivity disorder (ADHD). She brings up an interesting concept.

First, she notes that, through her research, she's talked to people who are microdosing psilocybin for ADHD. This makes sense since it has a slight stimulant effect. But that's not how she's used it. Instead, she's taken higher doses.

"Psilocybin's maybe been less helpful for ADHD," she says, "and really helpful for trauma. It allows me to reflect on my behavior and on my life and gives me insights into things that can be helpful for building the coping mechanisms I need around ADHD."

Having ADHD in an ableist world

Magic mushrooms are also helping Agro process wounds from childhood. "People with ADHD," she says, "most of us that I've met, have trauma as well because of having ADHD and being a disabled person in an ableist world that is not built for us."

She's careful and clear not to place blame on her parents when she speaks. "But being a kid with ADHD," she says, "you encounter adults around you who are just constantly frustrated and disappointed in you for being who you are—and you can't help it."

As a parent of a child who Agro says she's certain has ADHD (although not diagnosed yet), Agro recognizes the challenges. "It's like I'm time traveling back into my own parents' bodies," she says. She offers the example of auditory processing disorder, which is common with ADHD. "I have to say her name 10 times before she will look up at me," Agro says. "And it's not that she has an ear problem; it's that she's neurodivergent and she's focused on whatever she's doing."

Not every parent is as well versed in ADHD as Agro is, and not understanding a behavior can lead to frustration. Over time, outward displays of frustration toward a child—whether from a parent, a teacher, or another adult in their life—can breed shame within the child. That shame can turn into trauma. "Using psilocybin, for me," Agro says, "has been really, really healing because of a few things. One is that psilocybin, it gives you self-empathy. And it has helped me develop self-love."

To look in the mirror or not to: that is the question

If you've read up on psilocybin and some other psychedelics, you may have heard that you should avoid looking in a mirror. Well, several people I talked to for this book who have tried psilocybin, Agro included, have a story about looking in the mirror, and those instances turned out fine. (I did so myself. It was fine.) Agro says to just be prepared if you choose to look in the mirror and to not take the decision lightly. She says she was scared to do so because she was high AF. But doing so gave her a realization. "I remember being like, 'I'm so beautiful. I am a person,'" she recalls. "'I am just a human being with a face. And these eyes let me see. And this mouth lets me communicate and eat and keep myself alive. And how could I ever think badly about this face?'" She sums up her realization: "I am a person who's worthy of love. I am a person who's okay just the way I am."

Agro points out that psilocybin isn't the only thing that's helped her. She's also done work in therapy and tapped into other forms of support. "But it's been a really important tool in the tool kit for healing my relationship with myself."

Chapter 10

GIVE ME the Logistics

What are the best practices for using psilocybin?

The topic of best practices could take up a whole book. And you're in luck. A great one exists. Michelle Janikian wrote *Your Psilocybin Mushroom Companion*. Her book covers logistics in detail, more so than I have space to cover here. I'm interviewing her for this chapter, and I encourage you to grab a copy of her work. I'm also interviewing experienced psychedelic user and psychedelic coach Lana Pribic, host of the *Modern Psychedelics* podcast, which is another treasure trove of info.[192] And I'm reaching out to a study author who has researched predictors for positive trip experiences. My hope is that expertise from these women provide you with the framework for setting yourself up for the best trip possible—if a trip is your goal. In this chapter, you'll learn about set (your mindset) and setting (environment), trip sitting, navigating challenging experiences, and the importance of integrating your experience (and how to do so) after a magic mushroom journey. Plus, I'm including details on how to microdose. And finally, you may also be curious about the legal landscape of psychedelics.

What are set and setting?

We'd all like to have a good trip, whether we're going camping or taking magic mushrooms. Just as we can't control everything about camping (the weather, the bugs, a tent malfunction), we can't control everything about a psilocybin trip. But just as we can do everything in our power to ensure a smoother outdoor adventure (pack layers, use bug protection, and test that tent), we can take care to lay the groundwork for a better psilocybin trip.

Research shows that feeling prepared for the experience and comfortable in the environment and with the people you're around can help prevent a difficult psilocybin journey.[193] This care comes with the work of what's called set and setting.[194] The late Timothy Leary, PhD, a psychologist and psychedelic advocate and his colleagues (Ralph Metzner, PhD, and Richard Alpert, PhD, later known as Ram Das) wrote about it in their book (first published in 1964) *The Psychedelic Experience: A Manual Based on the Tibetan Book of the Dead.* "He was just a really smart psychologist," Janikian says of Leary, "putting words to a concept that we already do with a lot of things in our lives outside of psychedelics. Our mood and where we are [will] affect the experience that we have, no matter what it is." Janikian shares the example of going on a first date. If you're in a bad mood and you go to a sketched-out place, you'll likely have a subpar date. So we do what we can to set ourselves up for an optimal date by adjusting our mindset and going to a place where we'll hopefully feel chill. The same is true for a date with psychedelics. "Indigenous folks have been controlling their set and setting for centuries in their ceremonies," Janikian adds. She has some simple advice for applying set and setting to your own psilocybin experience. You're in a vulnerable, almost childlike state when you're on psilocybin. "You've got to think of yourself as a little kid," she explains. "How would you feel safe and comfortable?"

Think of set as mindset, which involves your intentions, expectations, personality, and level of preparation going into a trip. Then think of setting as the environment in which you'll be doing your trip, including where, who is around you, and even cultural influences or applications.

Set

You may be familiar with the concept of setting intentions if you've ever taken a yoga class. For example, at the start of a class or home practice session, I will often set the intention to let go of a specific stressor or to find acceptance for something I cannot change or control in my life. With psychedelics, the concept is similar but also different.

"Intention is one of those things that is a little misunderstood," Pribic says. "The way that I understand it is, the purpose of the intention is to connect with your purpose and reason for having this experience. It's to safeguard against going into this blindly or prematurely or without a care in the world." But she adds that people often confuse intention with expectation. Pribic advises setting an intention and then letting it go so that you're not holding too tightly to your preconceived notion of what you expect to get out of a psilocybin session.

"I think it's a little misguided sometimes to really set a lot of intentions," Janikian adds. "Instead, ask yourself why you're taking a psychedelic. Are you doing it to learn about yourself?" That's Janikian's general intention when using psilocybin. "Whenever I set really specific intentions, it can just be a bit heavy," she explains. "I can get too deep in thought loops about them and it kind of narrows my trip." She prefers to approach a trip with an open mind and let the mushroom teach or lead her.

These statements from Pribic and Janikian regarding set echo the results of a study in which researchers were trying to figure out if state of mind and personality help predict magic mushroom experience and outcomes. For the study, published in *Psychopharmacology* in 2019, researchers used crowdsourcing to survey 183 participants.[195] They asked them about their personality traits, state of mind, and life situation before ingesting psilocybin. They also asked them about their experience with magic mushrooms. The researchers found that willingness to surrender at the time of dosing was a strong predictor of having an optimal experience, and preoccupation was linked to adverse experiences. Their research replicated findings from their previous study, published in *Psychology of Consciousness* in 2019.[196]

The researchers describe surrender as a willingness to adapt to whatever unfolds during a psilocybin session, meaning releasing your preconceived notions, goals, habits, even the self. They describe preoccupation as being absorbed in your current life concerns or those of the past or future.[197] I reach out to Suzanne Russ, PhD, the lead author of both studies. She tells me that, although she didn't include this in the paper, the idea of surrender stems from the way Indigenous cultures have historically applied the use of psilocybin. "The rituals that would precede the ingestion," she explains, "would include things like fasting, or chanting, or other things designed to de-identify and to yield to the experience."

During a magic mushroom session, ego death (see Chapter Three) through psilocybin's effects on the brain's DMN serves as the catalyst for much of the psychedelic experience. "It's almost like one would precede that by stepping away already from identity," Russ says. Your set and setting preparation may involve practices that help you shed your sense of self, preconceived notions, and rigidity. When Russ was deep into the research on her studies, the movie *Frozen* was at its height of popularity. She says one of the people she spoke to during her research described the surrender like the character Elsa's experience. "When she finally let go and just let go of all her constraints," she explains. "It's that full release of everything you were." Or think of surrender as being willing to transition into something new. Some helpful tactics in the days leading up to your psilocybin journey or on the day of your trip may include eating lighter or fasting, abstaining from digital media, and even engaging in silence. "I think we have to deactivate our cognitive pathways and come into touch with more of our sensory experience," Russ says.

According to Russ's research, surrender is linked with positive experiences, while preoccupation is linked with adverse experiences on psilocybin.[198] Essentially, before a psilocybin experience, you want to clear your mind of your to-do list. Otherwise your mind is focused on what is forthcoming in this life, Russ says, and that is an inhibitor to an experience and even linked to unfavorable ones. Preoccupation may magnify, in a trip, whatever it is you're hyperfocused on, whether that's work, mundane tasks, or an upcoming event or deadline.

Russ offers a great way to think about the concept of releasing yourself from preoccupation. "If you're going to go to Mardi Gras or something like that," she says, "you have to release everything and put on your costume to go. You can't be holding on to all of the things that are going to be waiting for you afterwards." So, for a psilocybin trip, you must "remove your costume of this life," she adds. Instead, put on your I'm-going-to-try-psilocybin costume and adopt the open mindset of a child. You can't wear both costumes—your current-life one and your psilocybin one—at the same time. So how do you avoid preoccupation? Clear your schedule for your trip day. Allot plenty of time for the experience and for relaxing and considering your experience afterward.

We often think of set as a concept related to trip prep, but really, it's important throughout your psilocybin journey. And that's why I'm including another thing Russ notes: the idea of noble silence, a Buddhist philosophy or technique. It involves observing silence or only speaking necessary words. Such a technique may be helpful when you're on magic mushrooms or about to embark on your journey. "I wanted to look at whether talking during the experience would limit the experience," Russ explains, "because we're dealing with ineffable constructs, constructs that can't be put into words." She found that talking did predict negative experiences. "Not talking might be a beneficial thing," she says, "for accessing an experience that's transformational and beneficial to a person." But why? "Our thinking brain, our cognitive perspective," Russ explains, "is linked to our language. And language imposes a schema, a framework on our way of thinking that prevents us from seeing other ways." To further explain the concept, she describes the DMN as all that we've learned in our lifetime and all the pathways that lock us into default patterns of thinking. "Language has a really foundational impact on that," Russ adds. The temporary impacts to the DMN during a psilocybin trip allow for new ways of thinking, but language can hinder that process.

Setting

Setting involves where you'll physically be during a magic mushroom trip, but it's also about fine-tuning your environment for comfort, safety, ease, aesthetics, mood and vibe, and more. Plus, as Janikian notes, it's often closely related to set. For example, if her intention is to feel more in touch with nature, she might collect some seashells to use in her setting.

Both Janikian and Pribic mention that preparing an altar can be helpful. "I always go outside," Pribic says, "and forage for whatever I can find and put it on the altar. There will be a candle and some really grounding elements that can always be my anchor during the journey if I need to come back or ground myself." If Pribic is in a city setting, she'll close the blinds and curtains and cocoon herself from the outside world. She also puts her phone away to avoid distractions—after alerting a trusted friend to what she's doing. But setting is up to you. You might prepare a cozy space with pillows or create a relaxing playlist you can turn to if you decide you want music.

Ceremony can play a role in both your set and setting by easing you into the right mindset and adding to the aesthetics of your surroundings. "Having some kind of little ritual or prepping in some way," Janikian says, "really just helps prepare you and your mind for this big experience that's coming. It's like packing before you go on vacation. It's exciting and you are getting all the things ready you think you're going to need. I think you can do a similar thing for a mushroom trip or any kind of psychedelic experience to make it a little special."

You will find your own ways that speak to you of infusing ceremony into your experience. Pribic says it's about "just having ultimate reverence and gratitude for the mushrooms and for their consciousness."

For more info on set and setting, again, I highly recommend Janikian's book mentioned at the start of this chapter.[199] And Pribic has a checklist you can download, along with other free resources. You can find those on the *Modern Psychedelics* podcast website.[200]

What's a bad trip? And how do I get through one?

Challenges aren't necessarily bad. For this reason, some researchers and psilocybin users prefer to nix the term "bad trip" in favor of "challenging experience."[201] We can all think of challenging life situations in our past that have benefited us in some way—a bad breakup that opened a door for something better, a tough work project that dramatically boosted your knowledge base, a stressful time that imparted a valuable lesson, a brutal athletic endeavor, like a triathlon, that showed you your mettle.

Abigail Calder, MSc, the doctoral researcher I interviewed about neuroplasticity (see Chapter Three), has a great example about her mountaineering hobby. "If I'm honest," she says, "I'm usually not having fun while I'm doing it. It's scary, exhausting, and cold. But as soon as I'm safely down, it feels amazing to have climbed that mountain. I think challenging trips can sometimes be like that."

Of nearly 2,000 psilocybin users surveyed about their most psychologically challenging trip, 84 percent said they benefited from the experience.[202] Those survey results were published in the *Journal of Psychopharmacology* in 2016. Not only did many of the respondents benefit, 76 percent also reported an increase in well-being or life satisfaction from the event. And about 60 percent rated the experience as among their top 10 most psychologically meaningful. More than 30 percent rated it in their top five.

"People often describe the challenging trip as a learning experience," says Calder, who was not involved in the research.

"They feel that they learned something important or meaningful about themselves, although it may have been painful. Perhaps they could work through some difficult emotions and now feel lighter, or perhaps they discovered an unsuspected personal strength." Sometimes we are unaware of our own grit and personal tools. "Discovering that you are stronger than you thought can be very powerful," Calder adds. "Sometimes challenging trips can therefore activate people's mental resources."

That's not to say that a rough trip is no big deal. It can be. Sticking with her mountaineering example, Calder says, "I also don't forget: Not everyone comes back from the mountains unharmed and empowered. The same is true for challenging experiences on psychedelics."

The research on challenging trips found that 62 percent of respondents rated their psilocybin experience as among the top 10 most difficult experiences of their lives, 39 percent rated it among their top five, while 11 percent said it was indeed the single most difficult.[203]

"Most people in the psychedelic community know at least one person who has had a bad trip that negatively affected them for a long time," Calder says. "I hope we better learn how to support those people in the future."

What is a challenging trip experience? Researchers conducting an exploratory analysis, published in 2020 in the journal *PLoS One*, used software to analyze self-reported intense psilocybin experiences (detailed on an online platform) that led to a negative outcome.[204] A bad trip, according to their research, typically involves paranoia, fear, anxiety, racing thoughts, and a sense of losing one's mind. Ego death and hallucinations are also common characteristics noted in other research.[205] (Of course, ego death is associated with positive experiences too.) The analysis was exploratory, so it cannot be taken as cause and effect. But the researchers also found a possible association with negative experiences when other substances were combined with psilocybin, when high doses of psilocybin were consumed, and when multiple doses of psilocybin were consumed in the same setting.[206]

During a psilocybin journey, you may encounter your "shadow," which could lead to a challenging part of a trip, or it may be just fine. Either way, you can get through it.[207] In her book, Janikian describes the shadow, so I ask her about it. "The shadow," she says, "is originally a Jungian concept in psychology, which is like all the things in your personality that you kind of don't want to admit to." The late Ann Shulgin, known as the "matriarch of psychedelic-assisted therapy,"[208] discussed shadow work at the 2019 Women's Visionary Congress.[209] Although sometimes difficult, shadow work can be helpful. "I think it's a really healthy thing," Janikian says, "to have that level of self-reflection and realize when you're not living up to the version of yourself you want to be." The trick is to not judge yourself or beat yourself up regarding what you see with your shadow. "We can also be really hard on ourselves," she adds, "especially as women in Western culture having to be these ideal versions." Her advice is to have self-compassion. And mushrooms can help you do that. Then later, when you're not on mushrooms, you can infuse that compassion into the rest of your life.

The work of set and setting can help prepare you for navigating a challenging trip. "If you're not open to and ready to deal with challenging moments," Pribic says, "I would say that that's an indication that the mindset's not there yet." Or the time may not be right to trip.

Janikian, who lost a friend in the months prior to our interview, tells me she held off on a mushroom trip recently because she didn't think she was in the right headspace for it. "Now it's been weeks," she adds, "and I feel like maybe I'm getting closer to being ready and I have more distance and perspective."

Tough trips—or difficult sections of otherwise great trips—can be uncomfortable, like finding yourself on a carnival ride you dislike.

The annoying part: Once you're on the spinning ride at the fair, you can't get off. The same is true for a psilocybin trip. But just as a carnival ride is temporary, so is a bad trip. As long as you aren't having some unrelated medical emergency during a psilocybin journey, you will be okay. Once the psychedelic effects wear off, the negative symptoms you are experiencing should also dissipate. "There've been times where it was just really hard," Pribic says. "I had to just ride it out, and my mind went into some places that I wasn't ready for ... I made it through and I learned from it."

You're not simply at the mercy of the mushroom, however. You can tap into coping mechanisms to get you through a tough experience. The researchers who surveyed the people who had the bad experiences also asked them how they coped.[210] The strategies that were most successful included trying to calm the mind, changing location, making a bodily change, adjusting an aspect of the environment like music, changing who is around you, and asking for help from a friend. You shouldn't drive while under the influence of psilocybin, so if you need to change location, that might mean switching the room you're in or changing from inside to outside. In terms of making a bodily change, that might include getting up and moving around, for example. Another analysis explored interviews with 50 people from Norway, most of whom had a challenging psychedelic trip.[211] The researchers gleaned from participants what they thought could be useful for navigating a rough patch. Tactics included meditating, focusing on breath, and not judging the situation.

You can also reach out to the Fireside Project's peer-support hotline (call or text 62-FIRESIDE) during or after a trip if you need someone to talk to about your experience.[212] If you want to speak to someone who is also BIPOC, transgender, or a military veteran, you can request to be paired with an "affinity peer volunteer."

What is integration?

Integration is the process of extracting and making sense of the lessons from your psilocybin experience and then implementing behavioral changes as you see fit. While the psilocybin experience expands your mind via the mechanisms and phenomena described in Chapter Three, integration after a trip is just as crucial. It's what you do with that mind expansion.

"I definitely walk away with some material to work with immediately after," Pribic explains, "but then it also continues to unfold throughout the weeks, throughout the months." She describes the work of integration as peeling through the layers to get at deeper meanings as time progresses.

You might integrate with just yourself and your journal, with a therapist who specializes in psychedelic integration, with a psychedelic coach (like Pribic), with like-minded friends who have experience with psychedelics, or with integration circles. Pribic says she's an advocate for creating community locally with an integration group. The benefit is that you'll be able to unpack your experience with people who also have similar experiences and who understand the complexities of psychedelic journeys, the language or jargon surrounding them, and the fact that they're often hard to put into words.

Bea Chan, of Sisters in Psychedelics, expresses the importance of finding integration circles where people share some of your lived experiences in this world.[213] "At SIP, we run monthly BIPOC sharing circles," she says. "Having somebody else from that cultural understanding come talk to you as you are integrating your journey and your medicine and your learnings is so important."

Janikian typically turns to journaling or talking through her experience with friends. She sums up integration as "just making space for it and thinking about it and engaging it in some way—

otherwise you're going to forget, and it's just going to become this crazy memory."

When planning for your psilocybin journey, arrange for some integration immediately after. Janikian says she also tries to schedule at least one day after a trip to pick apart the lessons learned. "There's this sense of an afterglow," she says, "which can be kind of nice. It's a mix of exhaustion and inspiration." She'll have a nice meal and spend time outside. "To just fully bask in the weird magical experience I just had," she adds.

Integration continues long after your experience—for as long as you keep thinking about your psilocybin journey and gleaning insights from it. And of course you may learn even more through a subsequent trip or microdosing.

What's the deal with dosing?

The lingo on dosing is a little different, depending on whom you ask and what species you're ingesting. But general ranges exist. The following rough ranges are based on *Psilocybe cubensis*, one of the more popular species, but experience can vary depending on the strain.

A microdose is 0.05 to 0.5 grams.[214] I discuss microdosing protocols in the next section. But in brief, with a microdose, you generally won't have noticeable effects like ego dissolution or visual distortions.

A mini or low dose is about 1 to 1.5 grams. With this dose, you will likely experience euphoria and heightened senses, like seeing colors more vividly.

A medium dose is around 1.75 to 2.5 grams. With this dose, you might notice some visual distortions along with more intense euphoria and some changes in perceptions, like fear extinction.

A high dose is 3 to 4 grams. With this dose, you are likely to experience ego death and oceanic boundlessness, and you may have a full-on mystical experience.

A "heroic dose" is 5 grams or more. The term was coined by Terence McKenna, an ethnobotanist.[215] With a heroic dose, you will likely experience a disconnect from reality via hallucinations, ego dissolution, and more. Mystical experiences often occur during a heroic dose.

What dose should you try? That's up to you. Janikian recommends starting low and going slow. "That's how I experiment with any new substance," she says.

Consider how well you're able to calm yourself and self-regulate. "If you're really scared and you have anxiety and you can't already self-regulate," Janikian says, "start low and see how it feels, because it gets really intense and scary and weird sometimes."

A 1-gram dose is a great way to get acquainted with psilocybin. You likely won't have a mystical experience, but you may feel some euphoria and gain confidence for ingesting a higher dose next time around.

Janikian's book starts out with her description of doing a high dose as a teenager, before she had all this knowledge about psychedelics.[216] "I did have a really deep experience that I don't regret," she tells me. "But I was unprepared for it in a lot of ways—totally emotionally but also logistically."

If you know that you're in a safe situation with safe people around you, a higher dose might feel appropriate to you. For example, if you're having a paid experience with a trusted trip sitter or a skilled psychedelic guide (like I did), you might feel more comfortable going deeper. In that case, a 3- to 3.5-gram dose might make sense.

Never feel pressured to go higher if you don't feel comfortable. And never feel pressured to take a heroic dose if you aren't ready. You can absolutely take baby steps when it comes to using psilocybin. I 100 percent encourage that.

What is microdosing and how do I do it?

Microdosing psilocybin involves regularly taking a small dose, one in which you do not have noticeable psychedelic effects—or they are quite minimal. People's goals surrounding microdosing run the gamut, from boosting mood to managing social anxiety to preventing migraine attacks. (See Chapter Eleven for the research thus far regarding psilocybin and these conditions.)

Several protocols exist for microdosing. One of the most popular is the Fadiman protocol, created by James Fadiman, PhD.[217] To follow this protocol, you microdose with 0.1 to 0.4 grams (dried) on days one and four, while abstaining on days two and three. You repeat for 10 cycles. Then you abstain for two to four weeks while evaluating how you feel before beginning again if it suits you. Microdosing every single day isn't recommended, because you will build up a tolerance.

Another popular protocol is the Stamets Stack, created by mycologist Paul Stamets.[218] If you follow the Stamets Stack, you'll microdose with not only psilocybin but also lion's mane (a non-psychedelic shroom) and niacin (vitamin B3)—hence the stack. I'm including the dosages *DoubleBlind* magazine provides for a 154-pound person.[219] For the psilocybin, the Stamets Stack includes a larger dose range of 0.1 to 1 gram (dried). At 1 gram though, and even anything around or above 0.5 grams, you'll likely notice some psychedelic effects. For the other ingredients, the Stamets Stack involves 5 to 20 grams of fresh lion's mane and about 100 to 200 milligrams of niacin.[220]

Niacin gets a disclaimer though. You should consult your healthcare provider before taking it. This is crucial if you have any medical conditions or take medications or other supplements; they could have niacin in them, and high doses of niacin may cause liver damage.[221] One other note about niacin is that it can cause skin flushing. The Stamets Stack also involves stacking the days you microdose. You'll dose for four days in a row and then abstain for the next three.[222] As with the Fadiman protocol, after several cycles, you might want to take a few weeks off to see how you feel.

What are best practices for trip sitting?

If you're planning on being a trip sitter for someone else, I highly recommend reading Janikian's book.[223] It features an entire chapter on trip sitting, along with the do's and don'ts.

One thing to consider is whether you feel safe with this person you've been asked to trip sit. Remember that they'll be in an altered state. Another is whether you have personal experience with psychedelics and can understand the mind-bending situation the person will be in.

If you've used psilocybin before, you'll be aware of how weird a trip can be and how sometimes things that are basic can feel profound, Janikian says. "You don't make your friend feel like an idiot for saying, 'Oh my god, the sky is blue,'" she explains.

Janikian says preschool teachers would make good trip sitters because of how psychedelics can put people in a vulnerable childlike state. With that in mind, she says, "Make them feel safe. Don't bring up the negative stuff. Don't dismiss what they're saying as worthless, stupid, or just the drugs talking." Instead, be warm and accepting, but also don't be condescending.

As a trip sitter, you're there to hold space for someone during their experience. "Be honest with yourself if you really can be there for them," Janikian says. "Can you handle your own emotions while they're going through really vulnerable ones?"

Pribic, who is trained as a coach and to hold space for people, has this advice: "I don't recommend people to do this if they don't know how to hold space for someone," she says. "Holding space is something that is completely selfless, and it's something that you have to take yourself completely out of, because it's a matter of just being present for someone else's experience without injecting yourself into it." Let their experience unfold as it will and be a shoulder as needed. "The medicine is the guiding energy in a psychedelic experience," Pribic adds, "and we don't want to interfere with that, because there's a process that unfolds during a psychedelic experience and a process that someone is going through. And if we inject ourselves into that, we might interrupt the process."

What about legality and access?

As I write this book, psilocybin isn't legal everywhere, and the legal landscape on psychedelics is rapidly changing. Two main terms come into play: legalization and decriminalization. In some countries, cities, and states, magic mushrooms have been decriminalized, generally meaning they are a low priority for law enforcement. But that doesn't mean they're legalized. In other places, psilocybin is legalized, or legalized only under specific circumstances, such as for medical or therapeutic use. The caveat here is that even if a substance is legalized somewhere, laws may still restrict aspects of sale or personal use, such as growing. But not always. Is your head spinning yet?

What I'm trying to make clear is that you need to research the laws wherever you intend to use, buy, or grow psilocybin. I can't incorporate the laws of every jurisdiction into this book or offer suggestions on access, because it would take up the entire book and such a book would be outdated in a matter of months.

Instead, I want to use this section to point out the need for decriminalization in the name of harm reduction. I reach out to the Multidisciplinary Association for Psychedelic Studies (MAPS) and secure an interview with Betty Aldworth, director of communications and marketing. MAPS, through the association's work regarding MDMA for the treatment of PTSD, has worked hard over the past three decades to educate the US Food and Drug Administration (FDA) and the US Drug Enforcement Administration (DEA) about psychedelics and their therapeutic uses. "We were absolutely the first to conduct psychedelic-assisted therapy research with the FDA," Aldworth says.

As of the writing of this book, under the Controlled Substances Act, psilocybin, MDMA, and LSD are classified as Schedule I drugs in the United States, meaning the DEA deems them to be "drugs with no currently accepted medical use and a high potential for abuse."[224] Well, flip to the next chapter, and you can see this classification is woefully outdated.

"An honest look at the science and an honest look at the criteria for the Controlled Substances Act," Aldworth says, "should mean that at some point—hopefully in our lifetimes—psilocybin is descheduled and is not controlled by the DEA any longer." This process might happen through a bill moving through Congress or through FDA approval of psilocybin as a treatment, which would then be a catalyst for other changes.

In 2018, the FDA granted "Breakthrough Therapy Designation" to COMPASS Pathways for psilocybin therapy for treatment-resistant depression.[225] The next year, the agency granted the same designation to the Usona Institute for psilocybin for the treatment of major depressive disorder.[226] The FDA grants this designation when a drug demonstrates in preliminary clinical trials that it may offer substantial benefit over existing therapies. As of the writing of this book, phase 3 clinical trials are now underway regarding magic mushrooms.

Ultimately the Controlled Substances Act is behind the times and is problematic. "The drug war and criminalization of people who use drugs," Aldworth explains, "has caused an immeasurable amount of trauma in the world. And the illegal status of drugs causes incredible direct harm."

Hilary Agro, an anthropologist and PhD candidate at the University of British Columbia, whom I interviewed for Chapters Eight, Nine, and Ten, has researched this topic. She tells me about the "Iron Law of Drug Prohibition," a term coined in the mid-80s by Richard Cowan, a cannabis activist.[227] She directs me to *Filter*, which has a great infographic, if you'd like to learn more.[228] Ultimately, prohibiting a drug doesn't make people use it less. That's been debunked over and over, Agro says, noting by way of example that people use drugs in prison. "When you prohibit a drug," Agro says, "all you do is incentivize people to be more careful about transporting it." She cites alcohol prohibition of the 1920s. All that did was encourage the creation of dangerous types of moonshine back in the day. And prohibition is why so many people are dying from fentanyl (and other synthetic opioid) overdoses nowadays.[229] "Fentanyl isn't a bad, evil, dangerous drug," Agro notes. "I was given fentanyl for my C-section in the hospital. It's an important drug. The reason it's in the supply is because it's way easier to transport." It's more potent than heroin.

Instead of the criminalization of drugs, Aldworth says we need harm-reduction strategies. Speaking in the context of psychedelics, she says pairing decriminalization with education for safe use helps. "We should be creating social, legal, and medical context where people can use psilocybin and reduce the risks," she says. Part of that framework involves educating people who might encounter people who use psychedelics; specifically, she mentions the need for first responders to have cultural training. "So they're able to help not harm when they're in the case of a psychedelic emergency," she explains, "which should be treated differently than most first-responder emergencies." MAPS has helped train first responders in Denver, Colorado.[230] An example of a psychedelic emergency might involve someone needing assistance to get through a difficult trip.

Decriminalization reduces stigma, which helps promote education and therefore risk reduction. When stigma is taken out of the equation, people feel safe to ask questions, learn more about psychedelics, access a safe supply, and seek out resources that foster best practices when it comes to use. That's what protects people—not criminalization.

Chapter 11

GIVE ME the Science

What do we know about psilocybin and women's health?

You can jump to any section using the subheadings to find the information you seek regarding psilocybin and conditions like premenstrual dysphoric disorder (PMDD), migraine and menstrual migraine, and more. Plus, you'll find a section on menopause symptoms. But first, here's a quick personal tale followed by some notes on how this monster chapter operates and a note on the importance of incorporating Indigenous wisdom as well as the findings from Western medicine.

A brief personal story

The day before I first found blood in my underwear at age 11, I was doubled over in the bathroom.

If this is what labor is like, I thought, *I'm never having kids.*

In my early teens, my ob-gyn eventually put me on oral contraceptives for period pain. And that was that. I spent a decade assuming all people with a uterus endured such pain and that I needed to suck it up.

Then at age 21, I was working as a television reporter on assignment covering the governor's race in North Dakota. The night before the election, I hid from my colleagues in a diner bathroom, bracing myself against the stall door, breathing through each plunge and twist of the invisible knife in my abdomen. Somehow, I made it through my reporting assignment.

That week, at the urging of my mom, I booked an appointment with my ob-gyn. He told me I likely had endometriosis and scheduled me for a laparoscopy to confirm the diagnosis and to remove the suspected endometrial growths. After the diagnosis and surgery, I still endured excruciating pelvic pain, so I went back to the doctor.

His advice: get pregnant. That would stop me from menstruating.

He left out the word "temporarily."

What was I supposed to do? Churn out babies for the rest of my reproductive years?

Sadly, his callousness and dismissiveness are all too common. Plenty of people just like me have been told the same thing—or worse. A different doctor later told me the pain was all in my head, despite the multiple surgical reports proving otherwise.

In the years that followed my first laparoscopy, I had four more to remove endometrial growths. None of those procedures brought me pain relief. Endometrial tissue kept growing in places it shouldn't, threatening to create more pelvic adhesions and complications. I tried every potential treatment and alternative remedy I could. I won't list them all, but they included taking a medication that would put me into medical menopause, having pelvic nerves cut to interrupt pain signals, getting pelvic floor Botox, and—the most extreme—having a spinal cord stimulator temporarily implanted.

Fast-forward two decades from my diagnosis, and we still don't have a cure or effective treatments for endometriosis, which, as I noted in the introduction of this book, affects 1 in 10 people of reproductive age who were assigned female at birth.[231] (Although extremely rare, people assigned male at birth can get endometriosis too.)[232] We probably won't have a cure anytime soon, considering the lack of research funding directed at the condition. The National Institutes of Health designated less than 0.1 percent of its health research funding for endometriosis in 2022.[233]

I share the trajectory of my chronic disease and the way the medical world sometimes treated me because it mirrors how many other women have been mistreated regarding chronic conditions. I didn't have a term for it two decades ago, but I do now: medical gaslighting.[234] Healthcare providers are more likely to brush off the symptoms of women (compared to those of men), tell them it's psychological, and misdiagnose them. Medical gaslighting also disproportionately harms people of color.[235]

Medical gaslighting is dangerous. It can lead people to question what they know about their own bodies. It can lead them to avoid or delay medical treatment, even in emergencies. I speak from experience. One summer morning in my late thirties, I woke up with a swollen arm. I brushed it off for an entire day, thinking I'd simply overdone it the past few days. I also felt silly for potentially having yet another thing wrong with my body. *Maybe it is all in my head*, I thought. But I knew it wasn't. When I finally landed in the emergency room, I learned I had deep vein thrombosis, a blood clot. Clots are a risk—albeit a low one—of using some types of hormonal contraceptives.[236] (Hormonal contraceptives, by the way, are often prescribed as treatment for endometriosis.) The situation could have resulted in a pulmonary embolism, which can be fatal.

I wrote an article, published in Healthline, about the signs those on birth control should watch for.[237] Since then, I've received a few messages (usually in the form of social media DMs) each year from women with varied symptoms, worried they also have a clot. I always urge them to go to the ER and get checked out.

In my case, treatment required an overnight stay, various intravenous meds, and then a three-month course of an anticoagulant. The amount of blood in my underwear was alarming to me as a child, so I was definitely not prepared for menstruation on blood thinners—especially with already heavy periods from endometriosis.

I wasn't alone in my alarm.

The other DMs I get are from people who bleed who've come across my article in a panicked search for an answer to their question: Am I hemorrhaging? You'd think that when prescribing blood thinners to someone who menstruates, a healthcare provider would warn them about the monthly crime scene they'll potentially see in the bathroom. Heavy bleeding affects 70 percent of those who get a period while on anticoagulants, yet it often goes undiagnosed.[238] It can result in anemia or other issues and may require treatment. I almost needed intravenous iron therapy, for example.

I share the clot story to further illustrate how the medical system sometimes bungles the care of people with a uterus—or those who once had one. Therefore, we often turn to each other—even total strangers online—for advice and support on how to manage the chronic conditions we grapple with that have inadequate treatments and a lack of research. We do this especially when we've been gaslit. I'm not saying that's the way it should be—only that it is. Finally, I don't want my statements to give the impression that I'm anti-medical establishment. I'm not. I'm a medical journalist, after all, with a staunch respect for research and science. I simply want to advocate for better care and consideration for all who enter the doctor's office.

How to use this chapter

I wish I could provide a plethora of evidence-based research on all sorts of conditions specific to those assigned female at birth and how psilocybin may be able to help ease symptoms. But research on female-specific conditions lags in the first place, so it also lags in psychedelic research. In this chapter I distill some of what we do know from research. I also attempt to connect some dots on what we know from preliminary or experimental research that holds potential for helping with some conditions. The caveat is that, before those dots can actually be traced in with marker, we need more research—and more specific research at that. For many conditions, scientists are still working to understand the targeted strategies for how psilocybin can help—if it can at all. I also include some anecdotal information from women who are using psilocybin to self-treat. None of this information should be taken as a substitute for medical advice.

The importance of Indigenous wisdom

Finally, before diving in, I want to note a concept that Natalie Villeneuve, MSW, RSW, brings to my attention: "Two-Eyed Seeing." Mi'kmaw Elder Albert Marshall of the Eskasoni First Nation brought the concept to the Western practices of mainstream science.[239]

"Essentially," Villeneuve says, "it's about being able to take the positive aspects of both the Western world and Indigenous world and blend them. You're recognizing that Indigenous knowledge has a lot of value and that Western knowledge has a lot of value."

Before Westerners even knew about magic mushrooms, Indigenous people had been using psilocybin for thousands of years.[240] "Worldwide, there are Indigenous populations who have different ceremonial uses of different psychedelic substances," Villeneuve says. "I'm generalizing when I say this, but so many of them have knowledge about how we can use these safely that we should be considering."

Right now, Western medicine is engaging in Western practices of studying psychedelics, but that's not the only knowledge base. "I think there's so much Indigenous knowledge that we are just not paying attention to because we're not recognizing it as valuable," Villeneuve explains. "It's not considered to be scientific, even though it actually really is."

The historical use of psilocybin and other psychedelics does present evidence. "Science is really about doing something over and over," Villeneuve says, "and seeing what results you get from it and then learning how to apply that." In many ways, Indigenous cultures have done just that. "Just because it's not in an academic paper or tested in the ways that are considered to be science," Villeneuve adds, "it's just often discounted, which is really unfortunate because we're missing a huge part of the picture because of that." However, she cautions that she does not want to see the Western world exploit Indigenous practices. Instead, the Two-Eyed Seeing concept can be helpful.

To incorporate the Two-Eyed Seeing concept into this chapter, I also consult Mikaela de la Myco, who focuses on womb care and healing facilitation in the Ma'at tradition. She grew up in a multicultural, first-generation Italian, Afro-Caribbean, and Indigenous Mexican family who lived in Los Angeles (occupied Tongva territory).

Does psilocybin affect women differently?

The answer is *maybe*. When researching the topic of challenging trips, I come across something interesting. An exploratory analysis found that challenging trip reports were more common in females. Although more research is needed, the analysis suggests that people assigned female at birth may experience psilocybin (even at similar doses) differently because of hormonal, enzymatic, and social differences.[241]

We do know that estrogen levels impact binding at $5\text{-}HT_{2A}$ receptor sites.[242] In an article for *Psychedelic Science Review*, former editor and one of the founders of the publication, Barbara E. Bauer, MS, synthesized some of the research surrounding this receptor. As a reminder, psilocybin and psilocin are $5\text{-}HT_{2A}/5\text{-}HT_{1A}$ receptor agonists. That means psilocybin binds to these serotonin receptors. Bauer notes that estrogen boosts the density of the brain's $5\text{-}HT_{2A}$ binding sites, notably in areas that control mood and emotion. She further notes that other findings related to how hormones impact serotonin receptors may have implications for an entourage effect.

Do women have a unique entourage effect?

Psilocybin and psilocin are not the only compounds, or alkaloids, in magic mushrooms. And remember, nearly 200 different species of *Psilocybe* exist, some with multiple strains. Think of each of these as a different recipe with varying ingredients—or alkaloids. Other magic mushroom alkaloids include norbaeocystin, baeocystin, norpsilocin, and aeruginascin.[243] The theory of the entourage effect is that different compounds may work in concert to produce a certain result. Research is still ongoing regarding the potential entourage effect with magic mushrooms and how we may be able to use it to our advantage. For example, is it possible that combining two strains produces a better trip? Again, more research is needed. What Bauer is pointing out is that sex hormones may play a role as well in how psilocybin affects us.[244] Do sex hormones and their unique trajectory in the context of the female reproductive system produce an entourage effect?

Does psilocybin impact the menstrual cycle?

Again, the answer is *maybe*. We don't have robust scientific research on this yet.

While researching topics related to women's health, I reach out to Natalie Gukasyan, MD, at the Center for Psychedelic and Consciousness Research at Johns Hopkins University School of Medicine. My intent is to ask her about her work on psilocybin and eating disorders (a separate section in this chapter). That's when she tells me she's about to publish a case series on menstrual changes and psychedelics. She sends me the details via email, and I'm giddy over the fact that researchers are looking into this.

In her case series, coauthored with Sasha K. Narayan, MD, Gukasyan interviewed three women ages 27 to 34 about their cycles after psychedelic use. Two of the women used psilocybin, so I will focus on their reports.[245]

The first is a 27-year-old with premenstrual dysphoric disorder (PMDD) who ingested around 1.5 grams of dried psilocybin mushrooms when she was 26. Her period came eight days early. And she noted worse-than-usual cramps and mood swings. Later, the woman microdosed psilocybin and noted a benefit to functioning in the face of her PMDD symptoms, though she did not experience symptom improvement.[246]

Another woman featured in the case series, now 31, was 28 when she ingested chocolate that contained psilocybin and a component of ayahuasca, another psychedelic. This woman had experienced amenorrhea (an absence of a period) for five years. The morning after consuming the psychedelics, her period arrived, and she experienced normal cycles for the next three months before noticing some irregularity again. A year later, she was diagnosed with polycystic ovarian syndrome (PCOS).[247] Menstrual irregularity is a common symptom of the condition.[248] She used classic psychedelics again at least a dozen times at moderate to high doses and reported that a third of those instances likely influenced the early arrival of her period. After her PCOS diagnosis, she also reported microdosing magic mushrooms and that while doing so she experienced menstrual regularity.[249]

Gukasyan notes that all three women in the case study said their cycles came early after consuming psychedelics. Two also reported the reversal of amenorrhea. And one reported a return to menstrual regularity.[250]

What might be the mechanisms? The basics of the menstrual cycle can help us understand how psilocybin may impact it—or how the cycle may impact a trip. A cycle's hormonal fluctuations occur along the hypothalamic pituitary-gonadal (HPG) axis (sometimes referred to as HPO for ovaries) in a feedback loop where changes in levels signal what happens next.[251] The hormones involved include estrogens, progesterone, gonadotropin-releasing hormone (GnRH), luteinizing hormone (LH), follicle-stimulating hormone (FSH), and more.

Menstruation kicks off what's called the follicular phase. Estrogen starts out low during this phase, and slowly climbs, peaking just before or around ovulation. During the follicular phase, progesterone remains level and low. After ovulation, the luteal phase begins. Here, estrogen dips, forming a valley, before climbing to a gentle peak and then declining toward menses. Meanwhile, progesterone peaks for the first time of the cycle in the middle of the luteal phase and then falls toward menstruation. If you look at a chart of these hormonal fluctuations, they appear like a roller-coaster ride, and the changes around ovulation and in the luteal phase are often what cause premenstrual or other symptoms.

Now add psilocybin to the mix. Consider that psilocybin binds to serotonin receptors. Serotonin activates and regulates the hypothalamic-pituitary-adrenal (HPA) axis, a feedback system that regulates your stress response, among other things.[252] And the HPG axis (the one controlling the menstrual cycle) impacts the HPA axis.[253] In animal models, estradiol (estrogen) raises cortisol (stress hormone) levels, for example.[254] Likewise, evidence suggests that stress response can also impact sex hormone levels, illustrating that these closely intertwined axes affect each other,[255] though all the mechanisms of interplay still need much more study. Theoretically, a psilocybin journey or microdosing could impact the HPG axis and therefore affect your menstrual cycle. But we don't have definitive answers, just anecdotal reports and case studies that suggest a connection.

In their case series, Gukasyan and Narayan also note that classic psychedelics, including psilocybin, may directly or indirectly impact the menstrual cycle somewhere along the HPG axis. The authors suggest that research on the hormone prolactin and stress hormone levels, like cortisol, after psychedelic use may help us understand whether psychedelics are associated with menstrual changes and, if so, how. Some older research on prolactin levels and psychedelics exists, but it's mixed. We simply need newer research and more of it. Gukasyan and Narayan also note that studying levels of prostaglandins, estrogen, and progesterone after psychedelic use will also be helpful.[256]

I ask de la Myco about whether it matters during a cycle when we use psilocybin. "I find that when people journey while they're on their moon," she says, "say they're in one of the heavier bleeding stages and they're eating mushrooms, I find that the mushrooms can be very exhausting on the body." Often people fast or eat lighter on the day of a psilocybin journey. But in the days leading up to a bleed, de la Myco recommends focusing on nutrient intake. She abstains from doing deeper mushroom journeys right before or during menses and notes a time during the cycle that may be more optimal. "I find that the energy afforded to us during the ovulatory period," she says, "is very conducive and helpful to the mushroom experience."

Womb care tips

The term de la Myco uses in her practice is "mushWOMB consciousness." You can engage in mushWOMB consciousness as part of your self-care, whether you're experiencing a condition like endometriosis or PMDD (both discussed in the conditions section of this chapter) or you just want to be more in touch with, well, your womb.

"I absolutely love how tertiary and parallel and interwoven the mushroom system for healing is to the womb system for healing," de la Myco says. "And a lot of the practices and principles that are utilized in one can be utilized in another and vice versa." She goes on to say that anyone can approach their womb-care experiences through an entheogenic lens. "There's more than just symptoms there," de la Myco says, "there is a symbolic and spiritual core or root. As we kind of get at that root a little bit, then the symptoms can kind of change a little bit."

If you're considering microdosing psilocybin to help with symptoms, de la Myco recommends doing so as a preventive. Even if you start microdosing early in your cycle, you may not see the benefit until three cycles out, she says. "Although I do see a lot of benefit already in that cycle that comes directly after beginning a protocol," she explains, "I just like to be realistic with people and say, 'The seed that you're planting now will be ready to harvest in three months.'"

A key goal of mushWOMB consciousness involves reestablishing "a healthy bond in relationship to one's womb," de la Myco adds. For that reason, she encourages infusing other elements of self-care. In her practice, she offers services that include saying mantras, singing, engaging in movement, and more. On your own though, you can keep it simple until you establish your rituals. "It can also be just taking a bath and rubbing your womb," de la Myco says, "addressing your body as a being with a consciousness." Give it time and be patient. "Just like the mushroom experience is a journey," she says, "the womb-care journey is the same. It requires and asks us to be very curious and expect nothing and be a humble student."

Can psilocybin help with … ?

This section is an alphabetical list of conditions that disproportionately affect or solely affect people assigned female at birth—or they may affect them differently. Psilocybin is either being studied or is under consideration for study regarding these conditions. However, in some cases, psilocybin is being studied for a condition that can also be a symptom of another condition. For example, researchers are extensively studying psilocybin for depression, and depression can be a symptom of menopause. This is by no means an exhaustive list, and since we're amid a psychedelic research boom, new research will continue to emerge. For that reason, I'll provide updates where possible on my website and socials.

Alcohol use disorder

Alcohol use disorder (AUD) is a brain disorder. Over time, it can cause lasting changes in the brain that can make treatment efforts or recovery difficult.[257] More people assigned male at birth have AUD than those female at birth.[258] However, in the previous decade, the rates of AUD in women increased by 84 percent, a much higher rate than the 35 percent increase in men.[259] People assigned female at birth also have a higher risk of alcohol-related cancers, health complications, and conditions, and AUD can disrupt the menstrual cycle.[260]

Women often develop AUD at an earlier age than men.[261] And research shows a stronger association between anxiety and depression and early onset of drinking in girls ages 15 to 18 than in boys of the same age.[262] Research also demonstrates that sexual abuse, emotional abuse, and emotional neglect before adulthood are associated with higher rates of AUD in women than men.[263] Animal models show that ovarian hormones may also play a role in alcohol-seeking behavior.[264] Plus, women with consistently higher estrogen levels tend to have higher alcohol intake.[265] Finally, animal models indicate that drinking behavior changes throughout the menstrual cycle as hormone levels fluctuate.[266]

Can psilocybin help? A double-blind randomized clinical trial, with results published in *JAMA Psychiatry* in 2022, included 93 participants (almost half of them women), ages 25 to 65, in its final analysis.[267] All participants had an alcohol dependence diagnosis and were not currently receiving treatment for AUD. The researchers randomly assigned participants to either receive psilocybin or diphenhydramine (an antihistamine) in two separate eight-hour sessions spaced four weeks apart. All participants were offered 12 sessions of psychotherapy, as well.

The researchers found that the percentage of heavy-drinking days over 32 weeks was reduced in the group administered the psilocybin when compared to those administered the antihistamine as placebo. Those taking the psilocybin had 9.7 percent heavy-drinking days, while those taking the antihistamine had 23.6 percent heavy-drinking days. The results correlated to an 83 percent reduction in heavy drinking for the psilocybin group, compared to a 51 percent reduction for the antihistamine group. After eight months from their first dose, 48 percent of those in the psilocybin group had completely ceased drinking. That's compared to 24 percent in the antihistamine group. At 38 weeks, participants who received the antihistamine were offered psilocybin and additional therapy sessions.[268]

The study authors report that adverse events related to psilocybin "were mostly mild and self-limiting."[269] A limitation of the study is that participants would likely know the difference between a mushroom trip and the usual side effects from an antihistamine, and this could have created bias among participants. Another drawback is that the study participants had lower drinking intensity than those in other AUD clinical trials.

Albeit promising, this is just one small clinical trial, so more research is needed to figure out potential dosing strategies and other factors, including any differences across genders.

Anxiety

Anxiety is characterized by frequent, intense, and persistent worry or fear about everyday events or situations. The global prevalence of anxiety is more than 7 percent.[270] In the United States, people assigned female at birth are much more likely to develop an anxiety disorder throughout their life than those assigned male at birth.[271]

The lifetime prevalence for women is more than 30 percent and more than 19 percent for men.[272] Several different types of anxiety disorders exist, and most have a higher prevalence in women.[273]

Psilocybin shows promise for easing anxiety. A study published in *Frontiers in Psychiatry* in mid-2022 assessed anxiety in psilocybin retreat participants.[274] In the study, attendees completed questionnaires assessing trait anxiety and state anxiety before the psilocybin ceremony, the morning after, and at one-week follow-up. Trait anxiety is anxiety that is part of your personality, whereas state anxiety is anxiousness in a stressful situation. Not all participants completed all questionnaires. Overall, the researchers found an association with the psilocybin experience and a rapid and persisting (at least for a week) anti-anxiety effect. They correlate these changes with ego dissolution and lasting changes to the trait of neuroticism. Neuroticism—the tendency toward negative emotions and problems coping with stress—is a common trait in anxiety disorders. The researchers suggest that psilocybin helps to alter personality structures that promote anxiety.[275] This type of study has lots of limitations, of course, and more research is needed.

In a double-blind, randomized, crossover trial, psilocybin was shown to decrease depression and anxiety in patients with life-threatening cancer diagnoses. That research was published in the *Journal of Psychopharmacology* in 2016.[276] In the study, the researchers administered psilocybin to 51 cancer patients with anxiety, depression, or both. The participants either received a low dose (considered a placebo) or a higher dose. Then, five weeks apart, they crossed over in the study to receive whichever dose they hadn't had yet. Measures of depression, negative mood, anxiety, and death anxiety decreased. And measures of quality of life, meaning of life, and optimism increased. At six-month follow-up, about 80 percent of participants continued to show benefits. The measures were both self-rated and rated by clinicians. Researchers attribute some of the positive changes to the mystical-type experiences participants had in high-dose sessions.[277]

More research is needed on psilocybin's potential to help with anxiety and to look at different types of anxiety disorders and figure out specific strategies. But the evidence is certainly growing.

Dementia

Dementia affects an estimated 50 million people worldwide, with Alzheimer's disease accounting for at least half, if not more, of cases. In the United States and across Europe, approximately two-thirds of people diagnosed with dementia or Alzheimer's are women.[278] Researchers say one reason for this is that women often outlive men. But sex hormones and the changes that occur surrounding menopause—especially estrogen decline—may also play a role, since estrogen appears to have neuroprotective effects. Research shows a link between early menopause and early-onset dementia, for example.[279]

Scientists at Johns Hopkins University are working on a pilot study to see whether psilocybin has potential for improving symptoms of depression in people with mild cognitive impairment or early Alzheimer's disease. The estimated completion date for that trial is the end of 2023.[280]

In a 2020 mini review published in *Frontiers of Synaptic Neuroscience*, researchers noted that the 5-HT$_{2A}$ receptor is highly concentrated in brain regions vulnerable to dementia.[281] They also provided details on some reported cognitive benefits from microdosing psilocybin.

Much more research is needed to figure out if psilocybin should be part of a strategy for easing the burden of dementia, but at least research is underway.

Depression

Depression is a serious mood disorder that can greatly affect quality of life. In their lifetime, people assigned female at birth are about twice as likely to develop depression than people assigned male at birth.[282] Hormonal fluctuations may be a trigger, since people assigned female at birth often experience depression-related conditions like PMDD, menopause-related depression, and postpartum depression.[283]

In a phase 2b double-blind clinical trial, researchers randomly assigned 233 participants with treatment-resistant depression to three different groups, each receiving a different dosage of COMP360 psilocybin (a synthesized form) along with psychological support.[284] One group received 25 milligrams, another group received 10 milligrams, and a control group received 1 milligram. Over three weeks, one dose of 25 milligrams, but not 10 milligrams, of the COMP360 psilocybin reduced depression scores significantly more than 1 milligram. At three weeks, 29 percent of participants in the higher dose group were in remission from their depression, compared to 8 percent in the lowest dose group. However, the benefits tapered after 12 weeks, at which point just 20 percent of the participants in the 25-milligram group still showed a benefit.

Adverse events occurred in nearly three-quarters of participants. Symptoms included headache, nausea, and dizziness. And the study authors noted in the results, published in the *New England Journal of Medicine* in late 2022, "Suicidal ideation or behavior or self-injury occurred in all dose groups."[285] Of the 12 participants experiencing these serious adverse events, five were in the 25-milligram group, six were in the 10-milligram group, and one was in the control group.

More research is needed to see how to produce sustained benefits, prevent adverse events, and how to best use psilocybin (or synthesized forms) as a potential strategy in easing symptoms of depression.

Previous research from the Johns Hopkins Center for Psychedelic and Consciousness Research investigated psilocybin's effects on major depressive disorder. The results of the randomized clinical trial were published in *JAMA Psychiatry* in late 2020.[286] The proof-of-concept study included 24 participants (16 of them women) with major depressive disorder who were not currently taking antidepressants. In the study, 13 participants were randomly selected to receive psilocybin treatment right away, while 11 were randomly selected to receive psilocybin after an eight-week delay. The participants received two psilocybin doses scheduled two weeks apart along with psychotherapy lasting about five hours.[287]

The researchers assessed participants' depression scores via the GRID-Hamilton Depression Rating Scale at trial enrollment, one week after completing psilocybin treatment, and again at four weeks. On the scale, a score of 24 or higher indicates severe depression, whereas a 7 or less indicates no depression. At trial enrollment, participants had an average score of 23. At one week and at the four-week follow-up, the average score was 8. The group that waited for their magic mushroom doses did not show a decrease in their depression symptoms prior to receiving psilocybin treatment. Of all 24 participants, 67 percent showed a more than 50 percent decrease in their depression symptoms. At four weeks, 71 percent showed that same decrease. And at four weeks, 54 percent were in remission.[288]

In February of 2022, the Johns Hopkins researchers provided results from a follow-up study with those same participants. Those results, published in the *Journal of Psychopharmacology*, showed that 75 percent of participants had a treatment response to psilocybin and psychotherapy and that 58 percent were in remission from their depression at 12 months.[289] The study reported on safety outcomes, noting that no serious adverse events or self-injurious behavior occurred and suicidal ideation was low.

Eating disorders

Anorexia nervosa, bulimia nervosa, and binge eating disorder are the eating disorders most discussed. But others exist, including orthorexia (an obsession with healthy eating) and what's called other specified feeding or eating disorder, or OSFED (a disorder that doesn't meet strict criteria for anorexia or bulimia). This is not an exhaustive list. The National Eating Disorders Association (NEDA) provides descriptions of 11 eating disorders.[290]

Eating disorders can occur in anyone, but the prevalence is higher in people assigned female at birth. The overall lifetime prevalence of eating disorders in Western countries is nearly 2 percent, whereas the prevalence in females is just over 2.5 percent. However, those stats do not include all types of eating disorders.[291]

As of the writing of this book, researchers are studying psilocybin to see if it has potential to help with eating disorders. A journal article written by primary author Meg J. Spriggs, PhD, published in *Frontiers in Psychiatry* in 2021, details a pilot study protocol regarding psilocybin and anorexia nervosa that is underway at the Centre for Psychedelic Research, Imperial College London.[292] The clinical trial is scheduled for completion in 2024.[293] In the journal article, the study authors note that anorexia nervosa is the most fatal of all psychiatric conditions, with a quarter of deaths resulting from suicide. Some research suggests that abnormal serotonergic activity and reduced concentrations of BDNF may contribute to anorexia.[294] Psilocybin binds to serotonin receptors and enhances BDNF expression. Cognitive rigidity and emotional avoidance are also characteristics of anorexia. A psychedelic experience often positively impacts these traits.[295]

The Center for Psychedelic and Consciousness Research at Johns Hopkins School of Medicine is also conducting a clinical trial on psilocybin and anorexia nervosa.[296] "We are currently doing a preliminary analysis of the data, through about one month follow-up," Natalie Gukasyan, MD, tells me via email. "I can share that, on average, there seem to be modest but significant improvements in eating disorder symptom severity, quality of life, and depression scores between baseline and one month follow-up." She offers some caveats. One is that their intervention had a lot of flexibility with the number of sessions and time between follow-up sessions. The other is that the trial offered substantial psychotherapeutic support involving prep and integration. "With respect to adverse events," she adds, "this population generally has more medical and psychiatric complexity, and the types and amount of adverse events reflected that."

I ask her what the trial on anorexia nervosa tells us regarding other eating disorders and psilocybin. "We still have a ways to go with our understanding of two important unknowns related to this question: how exactly psychedelics work, and what the pathophysiology is of any of these disorders," she says. "Studies in people with bulimia and binge eating disorder have shown that other serotonergic drugs (namely common antidepressants) are superior to placebo, so it's possible that psilocybin could be effective via some serotonergic effect. Ultimately, we will need more research to determine if this treatment could be safe or effective for other indications."

Gukasyan and her colleagues recently published a review regarding psychedelic-assisted therapy and eating disorders and some hypotheses on the potential mechanisms.[297] Their review discusses the DMN (also covered in Chapter Three of this book). People with anorexia nervosa have increased resting-state functional connectivity between the DMN and the angular gyrus, which is part of the DMN. This increased connectivity is associated with issues regarding interoceptive awareness. Interoceptive awareness is our awareness of internal states of the body.[298] Psilocybin decreases resting-state functional connectivity of the DMN, which may provide a benefit.[299] Plus, psilocybin decreases amygdala reactivity, and Gukasyan and colleagues note this may be helpful for addressing "emotional reactivity to food and body-related cues," associated with anorexia.[300] Plus, psilocybin can help create what's called *psychological flexibility*, perhaps helping to encourage behavioral change. Psilocybin can also enhance openness, a common outcome when someone has a mystical experience. The openness and potential mystical experience may also facilitate behavioral change and enhance mood.[301]

If you haven't already, I encourage you to read Bridgette's story (Chapter Four) on healing from disordered eating, something she attributes to working with magic mushrooms.

Endometriosis and adenomyosis

Endometriosis is a chronic, systemic inflammatory pain condition. It causes endometrial-like tissue to implant and grow outside the uterus—leading to internal bleeding—often in the pelvic area.[302] (But it can also be found in unusual places, like the lungs.)[303] The lesions can then cause scar tissue adhesions that bind pelvic organs.[304] Adenomyosis is a related condition in which tissue similar to the uterine lining grows, often causing the uterus to enlarge.[305] Both conditions can be intensely painful, affect fertility, and greatly impact quality of life.

We don't yet have clinical trials that look at psilocybin as a potential to help ease symptoms of endometriosis or adenomyosis. But my eyebrows perk up anyway.

For one, we have anecdotal reports (as indicated in the section on menstruation) that psilocybin may play a role in regulating the menstrual cycle.[306] Irregularity is a common complaint of people who have endometriosis. Of course, we need more research on whether psilocybin can truly help with this.

Researchers are also looking at psilocybin for its potential to help ease chronic-pain. The research is just getting started.[307] A consideration is that psilocybin may have an anti-inflammatory effect. One study found that hot-water extracts from four psilocybin mushrooms downregulated pro-inflammatory mediators, known as cytokines, on human cell lines.[308] To be clear, this study was not conducted in actual humans, just on cells in a lab.

Cytokines are proteins that cells release, and they can either contribute to inflammation or reduce it. Pro-inflammatory cytokines—specifically interleukin-6 (IL-6), interleukin-1β (IL-1β), and tumor necrosis factor-α (TNF-α)—are involved in nociceptor sensory neurons that detect potential threats and lead to pain sensations, the study authors note.[309] Cyclooxygenase-2 (COX-2) is an enzyme also implicated in pain. In fact, non-steroidal anti-inflammatory (NSAID) medications inhibit COX-2.[310] Well, the magic mushroom extracts in the study, one of which included the popular Golden Teacher strain, significantly inhibited production of TNF-α and IL-1β, while also lowering concentrations of IL-6 and COX-2.[311] This experimental study did not research endometriosis or adenomyosis, however.

Consider this though. In addition to secreting hormones, endometriosis growths or lesions secrete pro-inflammatory cytokines.[312] They specifically secrete IL-6 and TNF-α, among others. Lesions are also known to increase COX-2 expression. And COX-2 overexpression is a risk factor for endometriosis recurrence after surgical removal.[313]

Again, we need more research before we can determine if psilocybin can help with chronic-pain from endometriosis or adenomyosis or how it might be used in combination with existing therapies. I just hope that research gets underway.

Fibromyalgia

Fibromyalgia is a chronic-pain condition that can affect the whole body. Symptoms might include tenderness, stiffness, brain fog, and sensitivity to light and noise. While the condition appears to affect more people assigned female at birth than those assigned male at birth, it may be underdiagnosed in men. It often goes undiagnosed or is misdiagnosed in general.[314] That may be because some medical professionals don't believe the condition exists.[315] (Gaslighting, anyone?) The World Health Organization recognizes fibromyalgia, as does the *International Classification of Diseases (ICD-10)*, and certainly the 2 percent to 4 percent of the population affected by fibromyalgia will staunchly tell you it exists.[316]

As of the writing of this book, researchers at the University of Alabama at Birmingham are planning an early clinical trial to look at whether psilocybin can help with chronic-pain, fatigue, and other symptoms associated with fibromyalgia.[317]

Additionally, researchers from the University of Michigan in Ann Arbor conducted a cross-sectional online survey asking people with fibromyalgia about their experiences with psychedelics.[318] Among the 354 participants, almost 30 percent had used psychedelics, with LSD and psilocybin the most popular choices. Fewer than 3 percent of those who used psychedelics for whatever purpose reported negative impacts on their health. Of 12 participants who used psychedelics with the intention of easing chronic-pain, 11 reported a benefit. The results of that survey were published in 2021 in the *Journal of Psychoactive Drugs*.[319]

Again, more research is needed on the topic, but I'm thrilled to learn that an early-stage clinical trial is in the works.

Menopause

Globally, about 47 million people assigned female at birth reach menopause per year.[320] Menopause occurs when your period has stopped for 12 months. For many, this milestone is naturally reached in one's early fifties.[321] But you may find yourself in natural menopause earlier. Induced menopause occurs for people who take certain medications (such as for cancer treatment) or who've had a bilateral oophorectomy (removal of both ovaries). In the years leading up to menopause, you'll be in perimenopause, also called the menopausal transition. This transition usually begins in one's late forties, but it could occur earlier. Perimenopause is apparent via changes in sex hormone levels that indicate declining ovarian reserve.[322] Your anti-mullerian hormone level is a good predictor of where you are on this trajectory, since it can be hard to gauge on your own.[323] You can ask your doctor for a test or order one online. You're in post-menopause once you've crossed the menopause threshold.

Perimenopause may be unnoticeable, especially in the early years of the transition. But it could eventually bring about burdensome symptoms that impact quality of life. These include hot flashes, depression, changes in libido, discomfort or pain during sex, mood changes, and insomnia or other issues with sleep. These symptoms can be so disrupting or frustrating that nearly 90 percent of women undergoing the menopausal transition or who have reached menopause seek guidance from their healthcare provider.[324]

During your reproductive years, the hormonal changes of your cycle occur along the HPG axis in a feedback loop. Perimenopause throws a wrench into that whole system. Hormonal changes in perimenopause can shorten your follicular phase, leading to earlier ovulation.[325] These factors can lead to extreme hormonal fluctuations that can drive the classic menopausal symptoms. At the time of menopause, estrogen levels will have declined by half, when compared to your reproductive years.[326] In post-menopause, progesterone is no longer produced.

Can psilocybin help with symptoms? I'd love to tell you I've come across definitive evidence. But as of the writing of this book, I'm not seeing studies or clinical trials on whether psilocybin can ease symptoms of menopause. However, we do have some evidence that psilocybin may be able to help with depression. Although more research is needed there as well, I want to focus on the depression aspect of menopause. The North American Menopause Society says people in perimenopause and in the early years of post-menopause seem to be particularly vulnerable to depression, likely because of hormonal shifts.[327] An older 2006 study found that women ages 36 to 45 who had no previous diagnosis of major depression in their premenopausal years were twice as likely to develop significant symptoms of depression in perimenopause than those who hadn't yet entered the transition.[328]

I contact Julie Freeman, who has her master's in counseling and psychology. She frequently works with women who are struggling with menopausal symptoms and who microdose psilocybin to help. She's held forums comparing psilocybin with SSRIs, which are often prescribed to treat menopausal depression. "With SSRIs," she says, "you can blunt the mood lability. So instead of having super highs and super lows, you can be kind of blunted. But it also blunts affect and it also blunts libido." Aye, there's the rub. "As a woman is going through menopause and estrogen declines," Freeman continues, "usually libido declines as well. That gets tied up in self-esteem. It's like 'My body's changing, my brain's changing, and now I don't even want to have sex.'" She notes the whole psychological domino effect that can occur. "Oxytocin is a chemical that's released during orgasm," she says, "and oxytocin is really important not only for mood and bonding and connection but it also plays a role in our brain health and our cardiovascular health." Psilocybin, however, may help address depression, but it does not further blunt libido as may occur with an SSRI, she adds.

In addition, psilocybin's 5-HT_{2A} receptor activation enhances the expression of BDNF. "BDNF plays such a role in our cardiovascular health and our bone health and our brain health," Freeman says. "Psilocybin—along with some of the other psychedelics—is known to help to improve BDNF. And while your SSRIs do as well, it seems like there's probably a better opportunity with psilocybin." Although low BDNF is implicated in depression, more research is needed to determine the association between BDNF levels and depression during the menopausal transition. Research indicates that progesterone and estrogen regulate BDNF levels and that BDNF is lower after menopause because of the decline in hormones, but fluctuating BDNF levels may play a role in mood changes during perimenopause.[329] Again, we need more research on this topic.

Freeman notes another way she sees psilocybin helping people during the menopausal transition. "Women will crave carbs and alcohol just as a way of trying to manage their feelings," she says. "One of the other benefits that's being looked at in the research with psilocybin is its ability to help with any kind of addictive tendencies."

An issue with the way women's health is approached is that doctors rarely consider the complete picture. Women's health has never really been taken seriously and "has never really been looked at from the totality of a woman's life," Freeman says. The whole picture is important, she notes, because of adverse childhood experiences (ACEs), explained in Chapter Eight. "Women who have ACEs," Freeman says, "are prone to having more challenges during perimenopause and maybe even into the menopausal years."

Higher childhood adversity scores are associated with more severe menopausal symptoms, according to results of a large cross-sectional study published in 2020.[330] Although the study doesn't tell us why there's a correlation, metabolic health may play a role, since ACEs can negatively impact metabolic health.[331]

Metabolic health is often defined as, without the use of medications, having ideal levels of blood sugar, cholesterol, triglycerides, and blood pressure, and having an optimal waist circumference. These biomarkers help signify optimal cellular functioning, which can help stave off chronic diseases. Worsening metabolic health, including high blood sugar and related insulin resistance, is associated with worsening menopausal symptoms.[332] By the way, the decline in estrogen toward menopause means we lose some of estrogen's protective effects against insulin resistance.[333] This is another potential reason for the increase in cravings Freeman mentions, and it may be a factor in menopausal weight gain. So to recap: ACEs can negatively impact metabolic health. Hormonal changes in menopause can also affect metabolic health. Researchers note a correlation between having more ACEs and more severe menopausal symptoms. They also see a correlation between worsening metabolic health and more intense menopausal symptoms. Taken together, we can see why a person's life history, rather than just their present health or situation, might matter when it comes to their menopause experience.

Freeman says she enjoys working with women in midlife because that is often when they're examining the big picture for themselves and considering how they want their life to look going forward. "There's a rebirthing process that's going on," she explains.

In a similar vein, de la Myco says, "A lot of women coming into their menopause time are in their wise-woman era." For that reason, a psilocybin journey can be synergistic. "What I really hope people can remember about the mushroom," de la Myco adds, "is that one of its original Indigenous applications was to teach a person what the meaning of their life was and why they came and why they were born." Psilocybin may be a catalyst for the reframing of how we think about menopause; we can treat the change as a rite of passage rather than something to be dreaded. "Mushrooms are absolute master teachers around transitionary phases," de la Myco says, "because they are decomposers. They help to literally transition one matter to another matter." This reframing of what menopause is—a transition—can help one tune into their feelings of self-worth. "When we get down to the purpose of our life," de la Myco adds, "then we can derive so much meaning."

I do want to add a word of caution when it comes to depression in midlife. People ages 45 to 54, across all genders, account for 80 percent of suicides in the United States.[334] And in Australia, women ages 45 to 54 had the highest suicide rates in 2015.[335] Having major depression increases the risk of suicide.[336] While we're seeing hyped and promising results from studies looking at psilocybin and depression, it's worth noting that suicidal ideation and self-injury have been reported as serious adverse events in psilocybin studies.[337] If you're experiencing depression related to menopause, it's worth consulting with a mental health professional. Seek immediate help if you're having thoughts of self-harm.

Migraine and menstrual migraine

Migraine, a debilitating and chronic neurological condition, affects those assigned female at birth three to four times more than it does those assigned male at birth.[338] Menstrual migraine, sometimes called hormonal migraine, involves attacks that occur just before or during one's period. Nearly two-thirds of women with migraine have menstrual migraine, according to the American Migraine Foundation.[339] The drop in estrogen right before menses triggers the attack.

Right now, we don't have robust clinical trials on whether psilocybin can help with migraine. However, a small exploratory study, conducted by Emmanuelle Schindler, MD, at the Yale School of Medicine, suggests that psilocybin has migraine-suppressing effects.[340] As a 5-HT_{2A} receptor agonist, psilocybin has some similarities to migraine treatment medications. In the double-blind, placebo-controlled, crossover study, researchers included 10 participants in the final analysis. Seven women and three men, all who had frequent migraine attacks, took a placebo capsule first. Two weeks later, they took a low dose of synthetic psilocybin. Over the course of the study, they kept a migraine symptom diary. The researchers found that the participants had a greater reduction of migraine frequency and pain intensity in the two weeks after the psilocybin dose when compared to the two weeks post-placebo.[341] Schindler is now conducting additional research to compare benefits of two psilocybin doses instead of just one.[342]

More research is needed to understand how and if psilocybin can work as a migraine prevention strategy and whether people with menstrual migraine might have similar results as those found in this small study.

Miscarriage grief

About 26 percent of all pregnancies end in spontaneous abortion, also known as miscarriage.[343] And 10 percent of people assigned female at birth will have a miscarriage in their lifetime.[344] About 44 pregnancy losses occur every minute worldwide. Pregnancy loss increases one's risk for anxiety, depression, PTSD, and suicide.[345]

I can't find any studies on psilocybin's potential to help people heal psychologically after a miscarriage. But we do have studies on psilocybin and depression, so it's not a stretch to consider that psilocybin may be able to help one cope after pregnancy loss.

I ask de la Myco about her experiences. She says she's sat in mushroom ceremony with several people who've turned to psilocybin as a way of introspection and transformation after miscarriage. She's clear, however, not to suggest that a psilocybin journey is somehow going to suddenly make someone feel completely better, regardless of their grief or trauma.

"Many people are actually left with more questions and more homework," she says. But those questions and the work done post-trip—such as with integration (explained in Chapter Ten)—can guide you. "Making sense of them in the thereafter," she says of mushroom experiences, "and doing the actions necessary in order to implement the mushrooms' teaching in their life is where that relief, the feelings of love, and the feelings of completion are going to come from."

Obsessive-compulsive disorder

Obsessive-compulsive disorder (OCD) is a chronic disorder in which people have uncontrollable thoughts or worries (obsessions) and behaviors (compulsions) that they repeat to lessen their obsessions.

For example, someone may engage in compulsive counting or other rituals to lessen intense anxiety.[346] OCD can greatly impact one's quality of life. The disorder affects about 1 percent of people, and those assigned female at birth are 1.6 times more likely to experience OCD than those assigned male at birth.[347]

Johns Hopkins University and Yale University both have clinical trials in the works to see if psilocybin can help ease the symptoms of OCD.[348] A 2006 pilot study from the University of Arizona, Tucson, investigated the effects of magic mushrooms on nine people with the disorder. The participants had up to four single-dose exposures (ranging in dose) of psilocybin. All participants had a marked reduction in their OCD symptoms. And no adverse effects occurred, aside from temporary high blood pressure in one participant.[349]

A paper in the *Journal of Psychedelic Studies* describes psilocybin's potential mechanisms that may be beneficial to people with OCD. Psilocybin may function as a "reset button" for dysfunctional activity of the brain's DMN that appears characteristic with the disorder.[350] More research is needed to determine if and how psilocybin can help.

Opioid use disorder

Opioid use disorder (OUD) is a psychiatric disorder. It is the dependence or addiction to opioids, the development of an opioid tolerance, and the presence of withdrawal symptoms when discontinuing opioids. More than 120,000 people die globally each year from OUD. And the condition affects more than 16 million people worldwide.[351] OUD can develop from the use of street drugs like heroin or from prescription drugs like oxycodone, or from both; prescription drugs are also sold illicitly. I recommend reading *Dopesick: Dealers, Doctors, and the Drug Company That Addicted America* by Beth Macy to gain a deep understanding of the complex issues that have fueled the opioid epidemic. Opioids have their place in patient care when it comes to acute and chronic-pain.[352] And drug policy changes and harm-reduction strategies are necessary to ensure safe access and safe use to people with OUD to prevent overdoses.[353]

While people assigned male at birth are more likely to die of an opioid overdose, overdose deaths in those assigned female at birth have been increasing. They've quadrupled since 1999 in the United States.[354] Women are more likely than men to have acute and chronic-pain and be prescribed opioids.[355] And they're more likely to report lifetime use, compared to men.[356]

A 2017 study published in the *Journal of Psychopharmacology* used data from the National Survey on Drug Use and Health (from 2008–2013) to determine if psychedelic use reduced past-year opioid use.[357] They looked at results from 44,000 illicit opioid users and found that psychedelic use was associated with 27 percent reduced risk of past-year opioid dependence and a 40 percent reduced risk in previous-year opioid abuse. Marijuana was also associated with a 55 percent reduced risk in past-year opioid abuse. But other than psychedelics and cannabis, no other illicit drug was associated with reduced risk surrounding OUD.

A study published in *Frontiers in Psychiatry* in 2020 looked at whether psychedelics were associated with a reduction in misuse of cannabis, opioids, and stimulants.[358] Of 444 survey respondents, 96 percent met substance use disorder criteria before their psychedelic experience. Only 27 percent met the criteria after. Most reported using LSD (43 percent) or psilocybin (29 percent).

Yet another study, this one published in *Scientific Reports* in 2022, looked at whether any lifetime use of classic psychedelics was associated with lower odds of OUD.[359] The researchers used data from the National Survey on Drug Use and Health (2015–2019), which featured nearly 215,000 respondents, with more than 2,000 who met criteria for OUD. They found that psilocybin was the only psychedelic associated with lower odds of OUD. The study has several limitations. The authors note that they cannot determine that psilocybin reduces the risk of OUD, only that there's an association. The same is true for all the studies mentioned.

The researchers of the 2022 study speculate that the effects magic mushrooms have on the serotonin system may play a role in resolving OUD. That's because abnormal serotonin transmission is associated with cravings and other aspects of addiction. Plus, mystical experiences may enhance recovery outcomes.[360]

The Johns Hopkins Center for Psychedelic and Consciousness Research is working on a clinical trial to investigate whether psilocybin administered in a supportive setting may reduce illicit opioid use. But that study will not be complete until sometime in 2024.[361]

Postpartum depression

About one in seven birthing parents develops postpartum depression (PPD), a serious psychiatric disorder that can occur after childbirth. But it often goes undiagnosed.[362] According to one study on treatment outcomes, only 6.3 percent of people with PPD receive adequate care.[363] Not only does PPD greatly impact the physical health and emotional well-being of the birthing parent, it can also impact the health, well-being, and development of their infant.[364] Plus, it can impact the child's future health and well-being.[365]

Scientists don't know the exact causes of PPD, but likely multiple factors play a role, including genetic, hormonal, psychological, and environmental.[366] Research indicates that people with PPD may be sensitive to changes in sex hormones. Low oxytocin levels may also be a factor. And evidence implicates HPA-axis dysfunction (which impacts stress response) and abnormal serotonin signaling as well.[367]

We don't have current studies on psilocybin and PPD, but researchers are interested. A paper published in mid-2022 in the

Journal of Psychopharmacology, coauthored by Chaitra Jairaj, PhD, outlines the potential for psilocybin to help.[368] PPD often involves a sense of isolation from others and a disconnection from both infant and self. Since psilocybin can enhance connectedness, perhaps this psychedelic or others may be able to help connect the birthing parent with their infant and facilitate connection with their support systems. Psilocybin may also help drive self-acceptance, which may aid in transcending the self-criticism that's a theme with PPD.[369]

You can find anecdotal reports online of people turning to magic mushrooms to cope with PPD. In a 2021 as-told-to article in *Good Housekeeping*, Melissa Lavasani describes the severe PPD she developed in 2017 and her experience with microdosing psilocybin.[370] And a 2019 *Vice* article by Maria Brus Pedersen (that originally appeared on the publication's Broadly Denmark channel) details author Julie Ugleholdt's experience with PPD and turning to magic mushrooms for help.[371] Ugleholdt also wrote a book on the topic entitled *In Project Baby—My First Year As a Less Than Perfect Mother.*[372]

Post-traumatic stress disorder

Post-traumatic stress disorder (PTSD) is a serious mental health condition that can occur in people who have directly experienced or witnessed a traumatic event. For a diagnosis, symptoms must last longer than a month. Symptoms include reexperiencing (such as having flashbacks), avoidance (such as avoiding thinking about the traumatic event), reactivity (such as being on edge), and cognition and mood issues (such as difficulty remembering the event).[373]

PTSD is a chronic condition that can be hard to treat. Only about one-third of patients recover within a year, and one-third remain symptomatic a decade after the trauma exposure. More than that, estimates show that up to half of people with PTSD who seek treatment do not have an adequate response.[374]

About 6 percent of people will experience PTSD at some point in their lives. People assigned female at birth have a two- to threefold higher risk of developing PTSD than those assigned male at birth. The lifetime prevalence for women is 10 percent or more.[375] The events most associated with PTSD in women are sexual assault and childhood sexual abuse.[376] Although more research is needed, traumatic stress may impact those assigned female at birth differently than those assigned male at birth. While males may have a more "physiological hyperarousal system," females may have a more sensitized HPA axis, at least according to animal models.[377]

A small clinical trial is underway to see if psilocybin may be able to help with PTSD.[378] But the results from that trial aren't ready as of the writing of this book. A paper published in mid-2022 in the journal *Cureus* highlights some of the potential that researchers see when it comes to magic mushrooms and PTSD.[379] PTSD is characterized by amygdala hyperactivity. But magic mushrooms, by downregulating the response to fearful stimuli, decrease that hyperactivity. In therapy then, possibly people with PTSD are more able to process trauma without having a trauma response. At the same time, psilocybin may boost mood, helping to reduce negative thoughts. Additionally, the paper authors note, the DMN is weakly connected and underactive in people with PTSD. The underactive DMN is linked to the avoidance symptom of the condition. Specific research on this is needed, but psilocybin's effects on the DMN may have positive effects for people with PTSD.[380]

Premenstrual dysphoric disorder

Premenstrual dysphoric disorder (PMDD) is a serious and severe form of premenstrual syndrome (PMS). Symptoms are often both physical and psychological. The physical symptoms may include cramping, vomiting, back pain, bloating, and more. And the psychological symptoms may include extreme irritability, depression, anxiety, trouble sleeping, feeling out of control, an inability to focus, and more. Symptoms typically occur one week before menstruation and end right before a period or a few days after it begins. As many as 8 percent of people assigned female at birth of reproductive age have PMDD.[381]

As of the writing of this book, I cannot find any clinical trials on psilocybin and PMDD. But this is another area where certainly the potential exists. Although researchers don't know the exact cause of PMDD, the serotonergic system has a close relationship with the hormonal changes of the menstrual cycle.[382] People with PMDD may be more sensitive to the roller-coaster ride of estrogen and progesterone levels.[383] Particularly, they may be more sensitive to those hormones' effects on the serotonergic system in the late luteal phase about a week before menstruation.[384] SSRIs, either taken continuously or only in the follicular phase of the menstrual cycle, are a treatment option for PMDD.[385] SSRIs work by blocking reabsorption of serotonin, making more of the neurotransmitter available in the brain.[386] But they can have unpleasant side effects.

Additionally, when they're in the luteal phase of the menstrual cycle, people with PMDD show increased amygdala response to negative stimuli when compared to people without PMDD. And in some cases, people with PMDD who have high trait anxiety also experience this heightened amygdala response in the follicular phase.[387] Although we don't have studies in people with PMDD specifically, we know that psilocybin reduces amygdala response to negative stimuli.[388]

Finally, in their case series mentioned in the menstruation section, Gukasyan and Narayan interviewed one woman with PMDD. Although microdosing psilocybin did not appear to reduce her symptoms, the woman credited the psychedelic with helping her function better despite those symptoms.[389] Again, we simply need more research.

Smoking cessation

Tobacco smoking rates vary globally. In the United States, more people assigned male at birth smoke than do those assigned female at birth. However, those assigned female are more vulnerable to the risks of smoking, such as lung and other cancers, cardiovascular disease and stroke, respiratory disease, and menstrual cycle disorders.[390] Nicotine impacts sex hormones and can lead to early menopause.[391] It blocks estrogen synthase in the brain, which could be why smoking cessation is also more difficult for women, according to research.[392] People assigned female at birth also have a difference in nicotine receptors when compared to those assigned male at birth, adding another reason as to why quitting may be trickier, considering most cessation methods focus on nicotine replacement.[393]

Psilocybin may be able to help. Johns Hopkins University conducted a small study with 15 participants (10 male) who were longtime smokers who had attempted to quit before but were not successful. After psilocybin administration during a 15-week cessation protocol that included cognitive behavioral therapy, the researchers found that 12 (80 percent) of the participants had ceased smoking at six-month follow-up. The participants were given two to three doses of 20 milligrams and 30 milligrams. The results of that study were published in the *Journal of Psychopharmacology* in 2014.[394] All 15 participants returned for a 12-month follow-up. At that time, 10 (67 percent) were smoking abstinent. At 16 months or more, only 12 participants had returned for long-term follow-up. At that time, 9 (60 percent) were smoking abstinent. The follow-up results were published in the *American Journal of Drug and Alcohol Abuse* in 2017.[395]

In a 2018 article in the *Journal of Psychopharmacology*, the researchers shared that participants in the pilot trial and follow-up were invited to participate in a follow-up interview 30 months after their psilocybin sessions. The 12 participants interviewed reported that their psilocybin sessions provided them with insight into why they smoked and that the content of their journeys outweighed any short-term withdrawal symptoms they experienced. They also noted persisting positive changes beyond that of quitting smoking.[396] More research is needed on the best strategies for using psilocybin for smoking cessation, but this small trial and follow-up seem promising.

Chapter 12

GIVE ME the History

What's the backstory on psilocybin and where do we go from here?

No book about psilocybin and women would be complete without the story of María Sabina Magdalena García, a Mazatec healer who lived in Huautla de Jiménez. The late María Sabina introduced white Americans to psilocybin mushrooms—albeit against her will.

"It's an example of how consent was broken," explains Natalie Villeneuve, MSW, RSW, whom I interviewed regarding consent in Chapter Six. "He lied to her to get access to this. That's not consent."

The man Villeneuve's referring to is the late Robert Gordon Wasson. He was a vice president at J.P. Morgan & Co. and an amateur mycologist. Feeling pressured, María Sabina agreed to let Wasson participate in a sacred ceremony and ingest the mushroom in the '50s.[397] But trickery was involved. "He said his son was missing," Villeneuve explains, "and he needed answers to find his son. That was not true." But part of their agreement was that he would not reveal María Sabina's name or location to anyone.

That agreement clearly meant nothing to Wasson, who went back to the United States and wrote about his experience in an article for *Life* magazine. In the article, he brags about being—along with the friend who accompanied him—"the first white men in recorded history to eat the divine mushrooms."[398]

"He essentially just gets really sloppy with covering up who and where she is," Villeneuve says. "What she consented to, or what agreement was made between them, he broke. So it's a violation of consent and it's an example of colonization, of how white people go in, claim something to be their own, take it to be something that it's not, and just exploit it."

As word spread, people from all over traveled to Huautla de Jiménez to try magic mushrooms. Famous folks, from Walt Disney to John Lennon, reportedly paid María Sabina a visit.[399] "The whole community," Villeneuve says, "really deteriorated as a result of tourists coming in and just not paying any respect to these practices." Once revered in her community, María Sabina was then blamed for the intrusion of Westerners. Her house was burned, her son was killed, and she eventually died in poverty, Villeneuve explains.

This is not a pretty story, and it's woefully short. By no means am I implying I've provided a complete history here—that would require a full book. However, I chose to end the book on this note because we're amid what's being referred to as a psychedelic renaissance. The research resurgence is exciting, but we must proceed with care not to do harm. I encourage you to follow the work of Psymposia, a nonprofit research and media organization that's serving as a watchdog for the psychedelic industry.[400]

As we move forward, we must hold accountable people who are using psychedelics to abuse power and violate others. We must consider the ways in which the pharmaceutical industry aims to capitalize on psychedelic substances and the impacts of that. We must consider the ways in which our use of psychedelic substances and psychedelic tourism impacts Indigenous people and their lands. Ultimately, our attempts to heal or have transformative experiences should not be at the expense of the well-being of others. Remember that psychedelics are great unifiers and not meant for self-gain.

ENDNOTES

1. Adam Winstock et al., "Global Drug Survey (GDS) 2020," accessed December 7, 2022, https://www.globaldrugsurvey.com/wp-content/uploads/2021/01/GDS2020 -Executive-Summary.pdf.

2. Miranda Olff, "Sex and Gender Differences in Post-Traumatic Stress Disorder: An Update," *European Journal of Psychotraumatology* 8 (2017), https://doi.org/10.1080 /20008198.2017.1351204.

3. Domingo Palacios-Ceña et al.,"Female Gender Is Associated with a Higher Prevalence of Chronic Neck Pain, Chronic Low Back Pain, and Migraine: Results of the Spanish National Health Survey, 2017," *Pain Medicine* 22, no. 2 (2020): 382–95, https://doi.org/10.1093/pm/pnaa368.

4. Lanlan Zhang et al., "Gender Biases in Estimation of Others' Pain," *The Journal of Pain* 22, no. 9 (2021): 1048–59, https://doi.org/10.1016/j.jpain.2021.03.001.

5. Anna C. Mastroianni and Ruth Faden, *Women and Health Research*, Washington, DC: National Academies Press, 1999.

6. Katherine A. Liu and Natalie A. DiPietro Mager, "Women's Involvement in Clinical Trials: Historical Perspective and Future Implications," *Pharmacy Practice* 14, no. 1 (2016): 708, https://doi.org/10.18549/pharmpract.2016.01.708.

7. Chloe E. Bird, "Underfunding of Research in Women's Health Issues Is the Biggest Missed Opportunity in Health Care," Rand.org, February 11, 2022, https://www.rand .org/blog/2022/02/underfunding-of-research-in-womens-health-issues-is.html.

8. Nanette K. Wenger, "You've Come a Long Way, Baby," *Circulation* 109, no. 5 (2004): 558–60, https://doi.org/10.1161/01.cir.0000117292.19349.d0.

9. Laura Hallam et al., "Does Journal Content in the Field of Women's Health Represent Women's Burden of Disease? A Review of Publications in 2010 and 2020," *Journal of Women's Health* 31, no. 5 (2022): 611–19, https://doi.org/10.1089/jwh.2021 .0425.

10. Krina T. Zondervan, Christian M. Becker, and Stacey A. Missmer, "Endometriosis," *New England Journal of Medicine* 382, no. 13 (2020): 1244–56, https://doi.org/10.1056 /nejmra1810764.

11. "Endometriosis," Yale Medicine, accessed December 7, 2022, https://www .yalemedicine.org/conditions/endometriosis.

12. Mitch Earleywine, Luna F. Ueno, Maha N. Mian, and Brianna R. Altman, "Cannabis-Induced Oceanic Boundlessness," *Journal of Psychopharmacology* 35, no. 7 (2021): 841–47, https://doi.org/10.1177/0269881121997099.

13. Henry Lowe et al., "The Therapeutic Potential of Psilocybin," *Molecules* 26, no. 10 (2021): 2948, https://doi.org/10.3390/molecules26102948.

14. Filip Tylš et al., "Sex Differences and Serotonergic Mechanisms in the Behavioural Effects of Psilocin," *Behavioural Pharmacology* 27, no. 4 (2016): 309–20, https://doi.org/10.1097/fbp.0000000000000198.

15. Alexander Lekhtman, "The Burgeoning Psychedelics Movement Still Excludes Women and People of Color," *Filter*, December 3, 2018, https://filtermag.org/the -burgeoning-psychedelics-movement-still-excludes-women-and-people-of-color.

16. Megan E. McCool, "Prevalence of Female Sexual Dysfunction among Premenopausal Women: A Systematic Review and Meta-Analysis of Observational Studies," *Sexual Medicine Reviews* 4, no. 3 (2016): 197–212, https://doi.org/10.1016/j .sxmr.2016.03.002.

17. Leah Moyle et al., "Pharmacosex: Reimagining Sex, Drugs and Enhancement," *International Journal of Drug Policy* 86 (2020), https://doi.org/10.1016/j.drugpo.2020 .102943.

18. Lily Kay Ross et al., *Cover Story: Power Trip, New York* magazine, 2021.

19. Lieke ten Brummelhuis and Jeffrey H. Greenhaus,"Research: When Juggling Work and Family, Women Offer More Emotional Support Than Men," *Harvard Business Review*, March 21, 2019, https://hbr.org/2019/03/research-when-juggling -work-and-family-women-offer-more-emotional-support-than-men.

20. Meredith Blackwell, "The Fungi: 1, 2, 3 … 5.1 Million Species?" *American Journal of Botany* 98, no. 3 (2011): 426–38, https://doi.org/10.3732/ajb.1000298.

21. Suzanne W. Simard et al., "Net Transfer of Carbon between Ectomycorrhizal Tree Species in the Field," *Nature* 388, no. 6642 (1997): 579–82, https://doi.org/10.1038 /41557.

22. Manuela Giovannetti et al., "At the Root of the Wood Wide Web," *Plant Signaling & Behavior* 1, no. 1 (2006): 1–5, https://doi.org/10.4161/psb.1.1.2277.

23. "A History of the Drug War," DrugPolicy.org, accessed December 7, 2022, https:// drugpolicy.org/issues/brief-history-drug-war.

24. Sarah Hughes, "American Monsters: Tabloid Media and the Satanic Panic, 1970–2000," *Journal of American Studies* 51, no. 3 (2016): 691–719, https://doi.org/10 .1017/s0021875816001298.

25. "Race and the Drug War," DrugPolicy.org, accessed December 7, 2022, https:// drugpolicy.org/issues/race-and-drug-war.

26. "Legal Marijuana Market Worth $102.2 Billion by 2030," GrandViewResearch.com, accessed December 7, 2022, https://www.grandviewresearch.com/press-release /global-legal-marijuana-market.

27. Megan U. Boyanton, "Entrepreneurs of Color Fight for Fair Share of Legal Weed Wealth," Bloomberg Law, November 30, 2021, https://news.bloomberglaw.com /banking-law/entrepreneurs-of-color-fight-for-fair-share-of-legal-weed-wealth.

28. Johannes Thrul and Albert Garcia-Romeu, "Whitewashing Psychedelics: Racial Equity in the Emerging Field of Psychedelic-Assisted Mental Health Research and Treatment," *Drugs: Education, Prevention and Policy* 28, no. 3 (2021): 211–14, https:// doi.org/10.1080/09687637.2021.1897331.

29. Roberto Lovato, "The Coming Psychedelic-Industrial Complex," Alta, January 4, 2022, https://www.altaonline.com/dispatches/a38326035/psychedelic-drugs -gentrification-roberto-lovato.

30. Grant Jones et al., "Associations between Classic Psychedelics and Opioid Use Disorder in a Nationally-Representative US Adult Sample," *Scientific Reports* 12, no. 1 (2022), https://doi.org/10.1038/s41598-022-08085-4.

31. "The Role of Purdue Pharma and the Sackler Family in the Opioid Epidemic," Govinfo.gov, US Government Publishing Office, December 17, 2020, https://www .govinfo.gov/content/pkg/CHRG-116hhrg43010/html/CHRG-116hhrg43010.htm.

32. Robert S. Gable, "The Toxicity of Recreational Drugs," *American Scientist* 94, no. 3 (2006): 206, https://www.americanscientist.org/article/the-toxicity-of-recreational -drugs.

33. Deborah Dowell, Tamera M. Haegerich, and Roger Chou, "CDC Guideline for Prescribing Opioids for Chronic Pain—United States, 2016," *MMWR Recomm Rep* 65, no. 1 (2022): 1–49, https://jamanetwork.com/journals/jama/article-abstract/2503508.

34. Michelle Janikian, "Types of Magic Mushrooms: 10 Shroom Strains You Should Know About," *DoubleBlind* magazine, last updated July 28, 2022, https:// doubleblindmag.com/mushrooms/types/psilocybe-cubensis-magic-mushrooms.

35. Ricardo Jorge Dinis-Oliveira, "Metabolism of Psilocybin and Psilocin: Clinical and Forensic Toxicological Relevance," *Drug Metabolism Reviews* 49, no. 1 (2017): 84–91, https://doi.org/10.1080/03602532.2016.1278228.

36. S. D. Muthukumaraswamy et al.,"Broadband Cortical Desynchronization Underlies the Human Psychedelic State," *Journal of Neuroscience* 33, no. 38 (2013): 15171–83, https://doi.org/10.1523/jneurosci.2063-13.2013.

37. Lukasz Smigielski, Milan Scheidegger, Michael Kometer, and Franz X. Vollenweider, "Psilocybin-Assisted Mindfulness Training Modulates Self-Consciousness and Brain Default Mode Network Connectivity with Lasting Effects," *NeuroImage* 196 (2019): 207–15, https://doi.org/10.1016/j.neuroimage.2019.04.009.

38. Gable, "Toxicity of Recreational Drugs."

39. Jones et al., "Associations Between Classic Psychedelics."

40. Rebecca Kronman, "Psychedelics and Pregnancy: A Look into the Safety, Research, and Legality," *Psychedelics Today*, October 13, 2022, https://www .psychedelicstoday.com/2021/09/29/psychedelics-and-pregnancy.

41. Lowe et al., "Therapeutic Potential of Psilocybin."

42. Frederick S. Barrett et al., "Emotions and Brain Function Are Altered Up to One Month after a Single High Dose of Psilocybin," *Scientific Reports* 10, no. 1 (2020), https://doi.org/10.1038/s41598-020-59282-y.

43. Dinis-Oliveira, "Metabolism of Psilocybin."

44. Barbara E. Bauer, "The Pharmacology of Psilocybin and Psilocin," *Psychedelic Science Review*, March 13, 2019, https://psychedelicreview.com/the-pharmacology -of-psilocybin-and-psilocin.

45. Jeremy Daniel and Margaret Haberman, "Clinical Potential of Psilocybin as a Treatment for Mental Health Conditions," *Mental Health Clinician* 7, no. 1 (2017): 24–28, https://doi.org/10.9740/mhc.2017.01.024.

46. David B. Yaden and Roland R. Griffiths,"The Subjective Effects of Psychedelics Are Necessary for Their Enduring Therapeutic Effects," *ACS Pharmacology & Translational Science* 4, no. 2 (2020): 568–72, https://doi.org/10.1021/acsptsci .0c00194.

47. R. R. Griffiths et al., "Mystical-Type Experiences Occasioned by Psilocybin Mediate the Attribution of Personal Meaning and Spiritual Significance 14 Months Later," *Journal of Psychopharmacology* 22, no. 6 (2008): 621–32, https://doi.org/10.1177/0269881108094300.

48. Theresa M. Carbonaro et al.,"Survey Study of Challenging Experiences after Ingesting Psilocybin Mushrooms: Acute and Enduring Positive and Negative Consequences," *Journal of Psychopharmacology* 30, no. 12 (2016): 1268–78, https://doi.org/10.1177/0269881116662634.

49. João Castelhano et al., "The Effects of Tryptamine Psychedelics in the Brain: A Meta-Analysis of Functional and Review of Molecular Imaging Studies," *Frontiers in Pharmacology* 12 (2021), https://doi.org/10.3389/fphar.2021.739053.

50. Bauer, "Pharmacology of Psilocybin."

51. R. L. Carhart-Harris and K. J. Friston, "REBUS and the Anarchic Brain: Toward a Unified Model of the Brain Action of Psychedelics," *Pharmacological Reviews* 71, no. 3 (2019): 316–44, https://doi.org/10.1124/pr.118.017160.

52. Karl Friston, "The Free-Energy Principle: A Unified Brain Theory?" *Nature Reviews Neuroscience* 11, no. 2 (2010): 127–38, https://doi.org/10.1038/nrn2787.

53. Robin L. Carhart-Harris et al., "The Entropic Brain: A Theory of Conscious States Informed by Neuroimaging Research with Psychedelic Drugs," *Frontiers in Human Neuroscience* 8 (2014), https://doi.org/10.3389/fnhum.2014.00020.

54. Carhart-Harris and Friston, "REBUS."

55. Carhart-Harris and Friston, "REBUS."

56. Carhart-Harris et al., "The Entropic Brain."

57. Carhart-Harris and Friston, "REBUS."

58. Abigail E. Calder and Gregor Hasler, "Towards an Understanding of Psychedelic-Induced Neuroplasticity," *Neuropsychopharmacology* 48 (2022): 104–112, https://doi.org/10.1038/s41386-022-01389-z.

59. Calder and Hasler, "Understanding of Psychedelic-Induced Neuroplasticity."

60. Calder and Hasler, "Understanding of Psychedelic-Induced Neuroplasticity."

61. David E. Olson, "Psychoplastogens: A Promising Class of Plasticity-Promoting Neurotherapeutics," *Journal of Experimental Neuroscience* 12 (2018), https://doi.org/10.1177/1179069518800508.

62. Cato M. de Vos, Natasha L. Mason, and Kim P. C. Kuypers, "Psychedelics and Neuroplasticity: A Systematic Review Unraveling the Biological Underpinnings of Psychedelics," *Frontiers in Psychiatry* 12 (2021), https://doi.org/10.3389/fpsyt.2021.724606.

63. N. L. Mason et al., "Me, Myself, Bye: Regional Alterations in Glutamate and the Experience of Ego Dissolution with Psilocybin," *Neuropsychopharmacology* 45, no. 12 (2020): 2003–11, https://doi.org/10.1038/s41386-020-0718-8.

64. Raphaël Millière, "Psychedelics, Meditation, and Self-Consciousness," *Frontiers in Psychology* 9 (2018), https://doi.org/10.3389/fpsyg.2018.01475.

65. Fengmei Fan et al., "Development of the Default-Mode Network during Childhood and Adolescence: A Longitudinal Resting-State FMRI Study," *NeuroImage* 226 (2021), https://doi.org/10.1016/j.neuroimage.2020.117581.

66. Damien A. Fair et al., "The Maturing Architecture of the Brain's Default Network," *Proceedings of the National Academy of Sciences* 105, no. 10 (2008): 4028–32, https://doi.org/10.1073/pnas.0800376105.

67. Carhart-Harris and Friston, "REBUS."

68. Alexander V. Lebedev et al.,"Finding the Self by Losing the Self: Neural Correlates of Ego-Dissolution under Psilocybin," *Human Brain Mapping* 36, no. 8 (2015): 3137–53, https://doi.org/10.1002/hbm.22833.

69. Mason et al., "Me, Myself, Bye."

70. Millière et al., "Psychedelics, Meditation, and Self-Consciousness."

71. Carhart-Harris and Friston, "REBUS."

72. Carhart-Harris and Friston, "REBUS."

73. Gaelle E. Doucet et al., "Transdiagnostic and Disease-Specific Abnormalities in the Default-Mode Network Hubs in Psychiatric Disorders: A Meta-Analysis of Resting -State Functional Imaging Studies," *European Psychiatry* 63, no. 1 (2020), https://doi.org/10.1192/j.eurpsy.2020.57.

74. Catherine I. V. Bird, Nadav L. Modlin, and James J. H. Rucker, "Psilocybin and MDMA for the Treatment of Trauma-Related Psychopathology," *International Review of Psychiatry* 33, no. 3 (2021): 229–49, https://doi.org/10.1080/09540261.2021.1919062.

75. Castelhano et al., "Effects of Tryptamine Psychedelics."

76. Bird, Modlin, and Rucker, "Psilocybin and MDMA."

77. Bheatrix Bienemann et al., "Self-Reported Negative Outcomes of Psilocybin Users: A Quantitative Textual Analysis," *PLOS ONE* 15, no. 2 (2020): e0229067, https://doi.org/10.1371/journal.pone.0229067.

78. C. J. Healy, "The Acute Effects of Classic Psychedelics on Memory in Humans," *Psychopharmacology* 238, no. 3 (2021): 639–53, https://doi.org/10.1007/s00213-020-05756-w.

79. Devon Stoliker, Gary F. Egan, Karl J. Friston, and Adeel Razi, "Neural Mechanisms and Psychology of Psychedelic Ego Dissolution," *Pharmacological Reviews* 74, no. 4 (2022): 874–915, https://doi.org/10.1124/pharmrev.121.000508.

80. Gregor Hasler, "Toward the 'Helioscope' Hypothesis of Psychedelic Therapy," *European Neuropsychopharmacology* 57 (2022): 118–19, https://doi.org/10.1016/j.euroneuro.2022.02.006.

81. Matthias Forstmann et al.,"Transformative Experience and Social Connectedness Mediate the Mood-Enhancing Effects of Psychedelic Use in Naturalistic Settings," *Proceedings of the National Academy of Sciences* 117, no. 5 (2020): 2338–46, https://doi.org/10.1073/pnas.1918477117.

82. Leor Roseman, David J. Nutt, and Robin L. Carhart-Harris, "Quality of Acute Psychedelic Experience Predicts Therapeutic Efficacy of Psilocybin for Treatment-Resistant Depression," *Frontiers in Pharmacology* 8 (2018). https://doi.org/10.3389/fphar.2017.00974.

83. Wanqing Li, Xiaoqin Mai, and Chao Liu, "The Default Mode Network and Social Understanding of Others: What Do Brain Connectivity Studies Tell Us," *Frontiers in Human Neuroscience* 8 (2014), https://doi.org/10.3389/fnhum.2014.00074.

84. Emily Blatchford, Stephen Bright, and Liam Engel, "Tripping over the Other: Could Psychedelics Increase Empathy?" *Journal of Psychedelic Studies* 4, no. 3 (2021): 163–70, https://doi.org/10.1556/2054.2020.00136.

85. Blatchford, Bright, and Engel, "Tripping over the Other."

86. Sisters in Psychedelics, accessed November 27, 2022, https://sistersinpsychedelics.org.

The PSILOCYBIN HANDBOOK for Women

87. Jiří Wackermann, Marc Wittmann, Felix Hasler, and Franz X. Vollenweider, "Effects of Varied Doses of Psilocybin on Time Interval Reproduction in Human Subjects," *Neuroscience Letters* 435, no. 1 (2008): 51–55, https://doi.org/10.1016/j.neulet.2008.02.006.

88. Katarina L. Shebloski and James M. Broadway, "Commentary: Effects of Psilocybin on Time Perception and Temporal Control of Behavior in Humans," *Frontiers in Psychology* 7 (2016), https://doi.org/10.3389/fpsyg.2016.00736.

89. Celina Timoszyk-Tomczak and Beata Bugajska, "Transcendent and Transcendental Time Perspective Inventory," *Frontiers in Psychology* 9 (2019), https://doi.org/10.3389/fpsyg.2018.02677.

90. N. L. Mason et al., "Spontaneous and Deliberate Creative Cognition during and after Psilocybin Exposure," *Translational Psychiatry* 11, no. 1 (2021), https://doi.org/10.1038/s41398-021-01335-5.

91. Mason et al., "Creative Cognition."

92. Mason et al., "Creative Cognition."

93. Mason et al., "Creative Cognition."

94. Frederick S. Barrett and Roland R. Griffiths, "Classic Hallucinogens and Mystical Experiences: Phenomenology and Neural Correlates," *Behavioral Neurobiology of Psychedelic Drugs* (2017): 393–430, https://doi.org/10.1007/7854_2017_474.

95. Kwonmok Ko, Gemma Knight, James J. Rucker, and Anthony J. Cleare, "Psychedelics, Mystical Experience, and Therapeutic Efficacy: A Systematic Review," *Frontiers in Psychiatry* 13 (2022), https://doi.org/10.3389/fpsyt.2022.917199.

96. Griffiths et al., "Mystical-Type Experiences."

97. Theresa M. Carbonaro, Matthew W. Johnson, Ethan Hurwitz, and Roland R. Griffiths, "Double-Blind Comparison of the Two Hallucinogens Psilocybin and Dextromethorphan: Similarities and Differences in Subjective Experiences," *Psychopharmacology* 235, no. 2 (2017): 521–34, https://doi.org/10.1007/s00213-017-4769-4.

98. Berit Brogaard, "Serotonergic Hyperactivity as a Potential Factor in Developmental, Acquired and Drug-Induced Synesthesia," *Frontiers in Human Neuroscience* 7 (2013), ahttps://doi.org/10.3389/fnhum.2013.00657.

99. Lowe et al., "Therapeutic Potential of Psilocybin."

100. Anna M. Becker et al., "Acute Effects of Psilocybin After Escitalopram or Placebo Pretreatment in a Randomized, Double-Blind, Placebo-Controlled, Crossover Study in Healthy Subjects," *Clinical Pharmacology & Therapeutics* 111, no. 4 (2021): 886–95, https://doi.org/10.1002/cpt.2487.

101. Carbonaro et al., "Psilocybin and Dextromethorphan."

102. Friederike Holze et al., "Direct Comparison of the Acute Effects of Lysergic Acid Diethylamide and Psilocybin in a Double-Blind Placebo-Controlled Study in Healthy Subjects," *Neuropsychopharmacology* 47, no. 6 (2022): 1180–87, https://doi.org/10.1038/s41386-022-01297-2.

103. Christopher W. Thomas et al., "Psilocin Acutely Alters Sleep-Wake Architecture and Cortical Brain Activity in Laboratory Mice," *Translational Psychiatry* 12, no. 1 (2022), https://doi.org/10.1038/s41398-022-01846-9.

104. Rylan S. Larsen and Jack Waters, "Neuromodulatory Correlates of Pupil Dilation," *Frontiers in Neural Circuits* 12 (2018), https://doi.org/10.3389/fncir.2018.00021.

105. J. E. C. Anthony, A. Winstock, J. A. Ferris, and D. J. Nutt, "Improved Colour Blindness Symptoms Associated with Recreational Psychedelic Use: Results from the Global Drug Survey 2017," *Drug Science, Policy, and Law* 6 (2020), https://doi.org/10.1177/2050324520942345.

106. Paul C. Bressloff et al., "What Geometric Visual Hallucinations Tell Us about the Visual Cortex," *Neural Computation* 14, no. 3 (2002): 473–91, https://doi.org/10.1162/089976602317250861.

107. Pantelis Leptourgos et al., "Hallucinations Under Psychedelics and in the Schizophrenia Spectrum: An Interdisciplinary and Multiscale Comparison," *Schizophrenia Bulletin* 46, no. 6 (2020): 1396–1408, https://doi.org/10.1093/schbul/sbaa117.

108. Brogaard, "Serotonergic Hyperactivity."

109. Anna M. Cabaj et al., "Serotonin Controls Initiation of Locomotion and Afferent Modulation of Coordination via 5-HT7 receptors in Adult Rats," *The Journal of Physiology* 595, no. 1 (2016): 301–20, https://doi.org/10.1113/jp272271.

110. Azad Ghuran and Jim Nolan, "The Cardiac Complications of Recreational Drug Use," *Western Journal of Medicine* 173, no. 6 (2000): 412–15, https://www.ncbi.nlm.nih.gov/pmc/articles/PMC1071198.

111. Dinesh K. Patel et al., "Mushroom-Derived Bioactive Molecules as Immunotherapeutic Agents: A Review." *Molecules* 26, no. 5 (2021): 1359, https://doi.org/10.3390/molecules26051359.

112. Maurizio G. Paoletti, Lorenzo Norberto, Roberta Damini, and Salvatore Musumeci, "Human Gastric Juice Contains Chitinase That Can Degrade Chitin," *Annals of Nutrition and Metabolism* 51, no. 3 (2007): 244–51, https://doi.org/10.1159/000104144.

113. Daniel Elieh Ali Komi, Lokesh Sharma, and Charles S. Dela Cruz, "Chitin and Its Effects on Inflammatory and Immune Responses," *Clinical Reviews in Allergy & Immunology* 54, no. 2 (2017): 213–23, https://doi.org/10.1007/s12016-017-8600-0.

114. K. P. C. Kuypers, "Psychedelic Medicine: The Biology Underlying the Persisting Psychedelic Effects," *Medical Hypotheses* 125 (2019): 21–24, https://doi.org/10.1016/j.mehy.2019.02.029.

115. Kuypers, "Psychedelic Medicine."

116. Thomas et al., "Psilocin Acutely Alters Sleep-Wake."

117. Lowe et al., "Therapeutic Potential of Psilocybin."

118. Carbonaro et al., "Challenging Experiences."

119. Ross et al., *Cover Story: Power Trip.*

120. Lowe et al., "Therapeutic Potential of Psilocybin."

121. Adam Winstock et al., "Global Drug Survey (GDS) 2021," accessed December 7, 2022, https://www.globaldrugsurvey.com/gds-2021.

122. Matthew W. Johnson, Roland R. Griffiths, Peter S. Hendricks, and Jack E. Henningfield, "The Abuse Potential of Medical Psilocybin According to the 8 Factors of the Controlled Substances Act," *Neuropharmacology* 142 (2018): 143–66, https://doi.org/10.1016/j.neuropharm.2018.05.012.

123. Ross et al., *Cover Story: Power Trip.*

124. Ross et al., *Cover Story: Power Trip.*

125. Lowe et al., "Therapeutic Potential of Psilocybin.

126. William E. Brandenburg and Karlee J. Ward, "Mushroom Poisoning Epidemiology in the United States," *Mycologia* 110, no. 4 (2018): 637–41, https://doi.org/10.1080/00275514.2018.1479561.

127. "Fireside Project," FiresideProject.org, accessed November 28, 2022. https://firesideproject.org.

128. Johnson and Griffiths, "Therapeutic Effects of Psilocybin."

129. Paul S. Appelbaum, "Psychedelic Research and the Real World," *Nature* 609, no. 7929 (2022): S95–S95, https://doi.org/10.1038/d41586-022-02875-6.

130. Jon E. Grant, "Psilocybin in Co-occuring Major Depressive Disorder and Borderline Personality Disorder," ClinicalTrials.gov, last updated August 5, 2022, https://clinicaltrials.gov/ct2/show/NCT05399498.

131. Michael Eisenstein, "The Psychedelic Escape from Depression," *Nature* 609, no. 7929 (2022): S87–S89, https://doi.org/10.1038/d41586-022-02872-9.

132. Lowe et al., "Therapeutic Potential of Psilocybin.

133. Dinis-Oliveira, "Metabolism of Psilocybin."

134. Emma I. Kopra et al., "Adverse Experiences Resulting in Emergency Medical Treatment Seeking Following the Use of Magic Mushrooms," *Journal of Psychopharmacology* 36, no. 8 (2022): 965–73, https://doi.org/10.1177/02698811221084063.

135. Lowe et al., "Therapeutic Potential of Psilocybin.

136. Melanie Flores, "SSRIs and Psilocybin Therapy: To Taper or Not," *Psychedelic Pharmacists Association.* December 19, 2021, https://psychedelicpharmacist.org/ssris-and-psilocybin-therapy-to-taper-or-not.

137. Aryan Sarparast, Kelan Thomas, Benjamin Malcolm, and Christopher S. Stauffer, "Drug-Drug Interactions between Psychiatric Medications and MDMA or Psilocybin: A Systematic Review," *Psychopharmacology* 239, no. 6 (2022): 1945–76, https://doi.org/10.1007/s00213-022-06083-y.

138. Sarparast et al., "Drug-Drug Interactions."

139. Flores, "SSRIs and Psilocybin Therapy."

140. American Psychiatric Association, *Diagnostic and Statistical Manual of Mental Disorders, Fifth Edition (DSM-5),* Washington, DC: American Psychiatric Publishing, 2013.

141. Pieter J. Vis, Anneke E. Goudriaan, Bastiaan C. ter Meulen, and Jan Dirk Blom, "On Perception and Consciousness in HPPD: A Systematic Review," *Frontiers in Neuroscience* 15 (2021), https://doi.org/10.3389/fnins.2021.675768.

142. Vis et al., "Perception and Consciousness in HPPD."

143. Pål-Ørjan Johansen and Teri Suzanne Krebs, "Psychedelics Not Linked to Mental Health Problems or Suicidal Behavior: A Population Study," *Journal of Psychopharmacology* 29, no. 3 (2015): 270–79, https://doi.org/10.1177/0269881114568039.

144. David Dupuis, "Psychedelics as Tools for Belief Transmission. Set, Setting, Suggestibility, and Persuasion in the Ritual Use of Hallucinogens," *Frontiers in Psychology* 12 (2021), https://doi.org/10.3389/fpsyg.2021.730031.

145. Ross et al., *Cover Story: Power Trip.*

146. "The 1 in 6 Statistic—Sexual Abuse and Assault of Boys and Men," 1in6.org, July 19, 2018, https://1in6.org/get-information/the-1-in-6-statistic.

147. Bianca D. M. Wilson and Ilan H. Meyer, "Nonbinary LGBTQ Adults in the United States," Williams Institute, June 1, 2022, https://williamsinstitute.law.ucla.edu/publications/nonbinary-lgbtq-adults-us.
148. Ross et al., *Cover Story: Power Trip.*
149. Forstmann et al., "Transformative Experience."
150. Caroline Hayes, Mourad Wahba, and Stuart Watson, "Will Psilocybin Lose Its Magic in the Clinical Setting?" *Therapeutic Advances in Psychopharmacology* 12 (2022), https://doi.org/10.1177/20451253221090822.
151. Hasler, "Toward the 'Helioscope' Hypothesis."
152. Sisters in Psychedelics, https://sistersinpsychedelics.org, accessed October 17, 2022.
153. Psychedelic Survivors, accessed November 12, 2022, https://www.psychedelic-survivors.com.
154. McCool et al., "Prevalence of Female Sexual Dysfunction."
155. Soheila Nazarpour et al., "The Association between Sexual Function and Body Image among Postmenopausal Women: A Cross-Sectional Study," *BMC Women's Health* 21, no. 1 (2021), https://doi.org/10.1186/s12905-021-01549-1.
156. "Sexual Health," World Health Organization, accessed November 12, 2022, https://www.who.int/health-topics/sexual-health#tab=tab_1.
157. Sheryl A. Kingsberg et al., "Female Sexual Health: Barriers to Optimal Outcomes and a Roadmap for Improved Patient–Clinician Communications," *Journal of Women's Health* 28, no. 4 (2019): 432–43, https://doi.org/10.1089/jwh.2018.7352.
158. Kingsberg et al., "Female Sexual Health: Barriers."
159. Helen E. O'Connell, Kalavampara V. Sanjeevan, and John M. Hutson, "Anatomy of the Clitoris," *Journal of Urology* 174, no. 4 (2005): 1189–95, https://doi.org/10.1097/01.ju.0000173639.38898.cd.
160. "FDA's Clinical, Statistical, and Biopharmacological Review of Viagra Clinical Development," US Food and Drug Administration, April 1, 1998, https://www.accessdata.fda.gov/drugsatfda_docs/NDA/98/viagra/viagra_toc.cfm.
161. Pugazhenthan Thangaraju, Hemasri Velmurugan, and Sree Sudha TY, "Drug Flibanserin–in Hypoactive Sexual Desire Disorder," *Gynecology and Obstetrics Clinical Medicine* 2, no. 2 (2022): 91–95, https://doi.org/10.1016/j.gocm.2022.04.003.
162. Rosemary Basson and Thea Gilks, "Women's Sexual Dysfunction Associated with Psychiatric Disorders and Their Treatment," *Women's Health* 14 (2018), https://doi.org/10.1177/1745506518762664.
163. Megan McCool-Myers et al., "Predictors of Female Sexual Dysfunction: A Systematic Review and Qualitative Analysis through Gender Inequality Paradigms," *BMC Women's Health* 18, no. 1 (2018), https://doi.org/10.1186/s12905-018-0602-4.
164. Sinan Tetik and Özden Yalçınkaya Alkar, "Vaginismus, Dyspareunia and Abuse History: A Systematic Review and Meta-Analysis," *The Journal of Sexual Medicine* 18, no. 9 (2021): 1555–70, https://doi.org/10.1016/j.jsxm.2021.07.004.
165. Emily R. Dworkin, Anna E. Jaffe, Michele Bedard-Gilligan, and Skye Fitzpatrick, "PTSD in the Year Following Sexual Assault: A Meta-Analysis of Prospective Studies," *Trauma, Violence, & Abuse* (2021), https://doi.org/10.1177/15248380211032213.
166. Lauren Gravitz, "Hope That Psychedelic Drugs Can Erase Trauma," *Nature* 609, no. 7929 (2022), https://doi.org/10.1038/d41586-022-02870-x.

The PSILOCYBIN HANDBOOK for Women

167. Gosia Phillips, "Investigating the Therapeutic Effects of Psilocybin in Treatment-Resistant Post-Traumatic Stress Disorder," ClinicalTrials.gov, last updated December 7, 2022, https://clinicaltrials.gov/ct2/show/NCT05243329.

168. McCool-Myers et al., "Predictors of Female Sexual Dysfunction."

169. Michele Ross, "Sex on Magic Mushrooms: Is It Safe?" Dr.MicheleRoss.com, last updated March 5, 2022, https://www.drmicheleross.com/sex-on-magic-mushrooms.

170. "Sexual Assault Statutes in the United States Chart," National District Attorneys Association, 2016, https://ndaa.org/wp-content/uploads/sexual-assault-chart.pdf.

171. "Plant Parenthood," accessed November 27, 2022, https://www.plantph.com.

172. Kronman, "Psychedelics and Pregnancy."

173. Kronman, "Psychedelics and Pregnancy."

174. The American College of Obstetrics and Gynecologists, "Committee Opinion: Marijuana Use during Pregnancy and Lactation," ACOG, July 2015, https://www.acog.org/clinical/clinical-guidance/committee-opinion/articles/2017/10/marijuana-use-during-pregnancy-and-lactation.

175. The American College of Obstetrics and Gynecologists, "Alcohol Abuse and Other Substance Use Disorders: Ethical Issues in Obstetric and Gynecologic Practice," ACOG, June 2015, https://www.acog.org/clinical/clinical-guidance/committee-opinion/articles/2015/06/alcohol-abuse-and-other-substance-use-disorders-ethical-issues-in-obstetric-and-gynecologic-practice.

176. Kayla N. Anderson et al., "ADHD Medication Use during Pregnancy and Risk for Selected Birth Defects: National Birth Defects Prevention Study, 1998-2011," *Journal of Attention Disorders* 24, no. 3 (2018): 479–89, https://doi.org/10.1177/1087054718759753.

177. Alana Rogers et al., "Association between Maternal Perinatal Depression and Anxiety and Child and Adolescent Development," *JAMA Pediatrics* 174, no. 11 (2020): 1082, https://doi.org/10.1001/jamapediatrics.2020.2910.

178. "Psychedelics & Maternity from Sex and Conception to Parenthood," *DoubleBlind* magazine, October 31, 2022, https://doubleblindmag.com/courses/psychedelics-maternity.

179. Barrett et al., "Emotions and Brain Function."

180. Jericho Hallare and Valerie Gerriets, "Half Life," In Stat Pearls, Treasure Island, FL: StatPearls Publishing, 2022, https://www.ncbi.nlm.nih.gov/books/NBK554498.

181. Thomas W. Hale, "Drug Entry into Human Milk," Infantrisk.com, accessed December 7, 2022, https://www.infantrisk.com/content/drug-entry-human-milk.

182. Lowe et al., "Therapeutic Potential of Psilocybin."

183. Hilary Agro, "Hi. I'm Back," April 13, 2021, https://twitter.com/hilaryagro/status/1382002201757900808.

184. Lisa M. Christian, Jennifer E. Graham, David A. Padgett, Ronald Glaser, and Janice K. Kiecolt-Glaser, "Stress and Wound Healing," *Neuroimmunomodulation* 13, no. 5–6 (2006): 337–46, https://doi.org/10.1159/000104862.

185. "Adverse Childhood Experiences (ACEs)," Centers for Disease Control and Prevention, August 17, 2021, https://www.cdc.gov/policy/polaris/healthtopics/ace/index.html.

186. Adam Schickedanz et al., "Intergenerational Associations between Parents' and Children's Adverse Childhood Experience Scores," *Children* 8, no. 9 (2021): 747, https://doi.org/10.3390/children8090747.

187. Centers for Disease Control and Prevention, "Adverse Childhood Experiences."

188. Kawther N. Elsouri et al., "Psychoactive Drugs in the Management of Post Traumatic Stress Disorder: A Promising New Horizon," *Cureus*, 2022, https://doi.org /10.7759/cureus.25235.

189. Sisters in Psychedelics, https://sistersinpsychedelics.org.

190. Blatchford, Bright, and Engel, "Tripping Over the Other."

191. "Moms on Mushrooms," accessed November 12, 2022, https://www .momsonmushrooms.com.

192. Lana Pribic, *Modern Psychedelics*, 2021, https://modern psychedelics.net.

193. Eline C. H. M. Haijen et al., "Predicting Responses to Psychedelics: A Prospective Study," *Frontiers in Pharmacology* 9 (2018), https://doi.org/10.3389 /fphar.2018.00897.

194. Ido Hartogsohn, "Constructing Drug Effects: A History of Set and Setting," *Drug Science, Policy and Law* 3 (2017), https://doi.org/10.1177/2050324516683325.

195. Suzanne L. Russ, R. L. Carhart-Harris, G. Maruyama, and M. S. Elliott, "Replication and Extension of a Model Predicting Response to Psilocybin," *Psychopharmacology* 236, no. 11 (2019): 3221–30, https://doi.org/10.1007/s00213 -019-05279-z.

196. Suzanne L Russ, Robin L. Carhart-Harris, Geoffrey Maruyama, and Melody S. Elliott, "States and Traits Related to the Quality and Consequences of Psychedelic Experiences," *Psychology of Consciousness: Theory, Research, and Practice* 6, no. 1 (2019): 1–21, https://doi.org/10.1037/cns0000169.

197. Russ et al., "Predicting Response to Psilocybin."

198. Russ et al., "Predicting Response to Psilocybin."

199. Michelle Janikian, *Your Psilocybin Mushroom Companion: An Informative, Easy-to-Use Guide to Understanding Magic Mushrooms: From Tips and Trips to Microdosing and Psychedelic Therapy*, Berkeley, CA: Ulysses Press, 2019.

200. Pribic, *Modern Psychedelics*.

201. Liridona Gashi, Sveinung Sandberg, and Willy Pedersen, "Making 'Bad Trips' Good: How Users of Psychedelics Narratively Transform Challenging Trips into Valuable Experiences," *International Journal of Drug Policy* 87 (2021), https://doi .org/10.1016/j.drugpo.2020.102997.

202. Carbonaro et al., "Challenging Experiences after Ingesting."

203. Carbonaro et al., "Challenging Experiences after Ingesting."

204. Bienemann et al., "Self-Reported Negative Outcomes."

205. Gashi, Sandberg, and Pedersen, "Making 'Bad Trips' Good."

206. Bienemann et al., "Self-Reported Negative Outcomes."

207. Janikian, *Your Psilocybin Mushroom Companion*.

208. David Presti, "Ann Shulgin: Radiant Nexus of Psychedelic Community," *Berkeley Blog*, July 11, 2022, https://blogs.berkeley.edu/2022/07/11/ann-shulgin-radiant -nexus-of-psychedelic-community.

209. Ann Shulgin, "Women's Visionary Congress 2019," Sandbagger News, YouTube, 2019. https://www.youtube.com/watch?v=aOy9N5TugZA.

210. Carbonaro et al., "Challenging Experiences after Ingesting."

211. Gashi, Sandberg, and Pedersen, "Making 'Bad Trips' Good."

212. Fireside Project, https://firesideproject.org.

213. Sisters in Psychedelics, https://sistersinpsychedelics.org.

214. Federico Cavanna et al., "Microdosing with Psilocybin Mushrooms: A Double-Blind Placebo-Controlled Study," *Translational Psychiatry* 12, no. 1 (2022), https://doi.org/10.1038/s41398-022-02039-0.

215. Terence McKenna, "Terence McKenna—A Heroic Dose (Psychedelic Notes: Part 2)," Soul Synergy, YouTube, 2016, https://www.youtube.com/watch?v=2XCEcWfifRY.

216. Janikian, *Your Psilocybin Mushroom Companion.*

217. James Fadiman and Sophia Korb, "Microdosing Psychedelics," accessed November 24, 2022. https://microdosingpsychedelics.com.

218. Danielle Simone Brand, "Can Microdosing Really Change Your Brain?" *DoubleBlind* magazine, last updated January 12, 2022, https://doubleblindmag.com/stamets-stack.

219. Brand, "Can Microdosing Really Change."

220. Brand, "Can Microdosing Really Change."

221. Kenneth Leung et al., "Niacin-Induced Anicteric Microvesicular Steatotic Acute Liver Failure," *Hepatology Communications* 2, no. 11 (2018): 1293–98, https://doi.org/10.1002/hep4.1253.

222. Brand, "Can Microdosing Really Change."

223. Janikian, *Your Psilocybin Mushroom Companion.*

224. "Drug Scheduling," US Drug Enforcement Administration, accessed November 24, 2022, https://www.dea.gov/drug-information/drug-scheduling.

225. "COMPASS Pathways Receives FDA Breakthrough Therapy Designation for Psilocybin Therapy for Treatment-Resistant Depression," COMPASS Pathways, October 23, 2018, https://compasspathways.com/compass-pathways-receives-fda-breakthrough-therapy-designation-for-psilocybin-therapy-for-treatment-resistant-depression.

226. Usona Institute, "FDA Grants Breakthrough Therapy Designation to Usona Institute's Psilocybin Program for Major Depressive Disorder," Usona Institute, November 22, 2019, https://www.usonainstitute.org/press-release/fda-grants-breakthrough-therapy-designation-to-usona-institutes-psilocybin-program-for-major-depressive-disorder.

227. Richard C. Cowan, "How the Narcs Created Crack: A War against Ourselves," UNOV Library Catalogue, accessed November 24, 2022, https://unov.tind.io/record/8741.

228. Sarah Beller, "Infographic: The 'Iron Law of Prohibition,'" *Filter*, October 3, 2018, https://filtermag.org/infographic-the-iron-law-of-prohibition.

229. Aliza Cohen, Sheila P. Vakharia, Julie Netherland, and Kassandra Frederique, "How the War on Drugs Impacts Social Determinants of Health beyond the Criminal Legal System," *Annals of Medicine* 54, no. 1 (2022): 2024–38, https://doi.org/10.1080/07853890.2022.2100926.

230. Sara Gael and Bryan H. Lang, "MAPS Harm Reduction Department Initiates Psychedelic Response Training for Denver First Responders—Multidisciplinary Association for Psychedelic Studies," *MAPS Bulletin 2021* 31, no. 2 (2021), https://maps.org/news/bulletin/maps-harm-reduction-department-initiates-psychedelic-response-training-for-denver-first-responders.

231. Zondervan, Becker, and Missmer, "Endometriosis."

232. Fadi I. Jabr and Venk Mani, "An Unusual Cause of Abdominal Pain in a Male Patient: Endometriosis," *Avicenna Journal of Medicine* 4, no. 4 (2014): 99–101, https://doi.org/10.4103/2231-0770.140660.

233. Katherine Ellis, Deborah Munro, and Jennifer Clarke, "Endometriosis Is Undervalued: A Call to Action," *Frontiers in Global Women's Health* 3 (2022), https://doi.org/10.3389/fgwh.2022.902371.

234. Melinda Wenner Moyer, "Women Are Calling Out 'Medical Gaslighting,'" *New York Times*, March 28, 2022, https://www.nytimes.com/2022/03/28/well/live/gaslighting-doctors-patients-health.html.

235. Wenner Moyer, "Calling Out 'Medical Gaslighting.'"

236. "FDA Drug Safety Communication: Updated Information about the Risk of Blood Clots in Women Taking Birth Control Pills Containing Drospirenone," FDA, February 13, 2013, https://www.fda.gov/drugs/drug-safety-and-availability/fda-drug-safety-communication-updated-information-about-risk-blood-clots-women-taking-birth-control.

237. Jennifer Chesak, "The Blood Clot That Could Have Killed Me," Healthline, July 10, 2017, https://www.healthline.com/health/birth-control/blood-clot-risk.

238. Bethany Samuelson Bannow, "Management of Heavy Menstrual Bleeding on Anticoagulation," *Hematology* 2020, no. 1 (2020): 533–37, https://doi.org/10.1182/hematology.2020000138.

239. Cheryl Bartlett, Murdena Marshall, and Albert Marshall, "Two-Eyed Seeing and Other Lessons Learned within a Co-Learning Journey of Bringing Together Indigenous and Mainstream Knowledges and Ways of Knowing," *Journal of Environmental Studies and Sciences* 2, no. 4 (2012): 331–40, https://doi.org/10.1007/s13412-012-0086-8.

240. David E. Nichols, "Psilocybin: From Ancient Magic to Modern Medicine," *The Journal of Antibiotics* 73, no. 10 (2020): 679–86. https://doi.org/10.1038/s41429-020-0311-8.

241. Bienemann et al., "Self-Reported Negative Outcomes."

242. Barbara E. Bauer, "Female Hormones, 5-HT$_{2A}$ Receptors, and Psychedelics," *Psychedelic Science Review*, December 10, 2019, https://psychedelicreview.com/female-hormones-5-ht2a-receptors-and-psychedelics.

243. P. Chue, A. Andreiev, E. Bucuci, C. Els, and J. Chue, "A Review of Aeruginascin and Potential Entourage Effect in Hallucinogenic Mushrooms," *European Psychiatry* 65, no. S1 (2022): S885–S885, https://doi.org/10.1192/j.eurpsy.2022.2297.

244. Bauer, "Female Hormones."

245. Natalie Gukasyan and Sasha K. Narayan, "Menstrual Changes and Reversal of Amenorrhea Induced by Classic Psychedelics: A Case Series," *Journal of Psychoactive Drugs*, (2023): https://doi.org/10.1080/02791072.2022.2157350.

246. Gukasyan and Narayan, "Menstrual Changes."

247. Gukasyan and Narayan, "Menstrual Changes."

248. S. Livadas et al., "Menstrual Irregularities in PCOS. Does It Matter When It Starts?" *Experimental and Clinical Endocrinology & Diabetes* 119, no. 6 (2011): 334–37, https://doi.org/10.1055/s-0030-1269882.

249. Gukasyan and Narayan, "Menstrual Changes."

250. Gukasyan and Narayan, "Menstrual Changes."

251. Sasha Mikhael, Advaita Punjala-Patel, and Larisa Gavrilova-Jordan, "Hypothalamic-Pituitary-Ovarian Axis Disorders Impacting Female Fertility," *Biomedicines* 7, no. 1 (2019): 5, https://doi.org/10.3390/biomedicines7010005.

252. Timothy G. Dinan, "Serotonin and the Regulation of Hypothalamic-Pituitary -Adrenal Axis Function," *Life Sciences* 58, no. 20 (1996): 1683–94, https://doi.org/10.1016/0024-3205(96)00066-5.

253. Mario G. Oyola and Robert J. Handa, "Hypothalamic–Pituitary–Adrenal and Hypothalamic–Pituitary–Gonadal Axes: Sex Differences in Regulation of Stress Responsivity," *Stress* 20, no. 5 (2017): 476–94, https://doi.org/10.1080/10253890.2017.1369523.

254. Oyola and Handa, "Hypothalamic–Pituitary–Adrenal."

255. Belinda Pletzer, Eefje S. Poppelaars, Johannes Klackl, and Eva Jonas,"The Gonadal Response to Social Stress and Its Relationship to Cortisol," *Stress* 24, no. 6 (2021): 866–75, https://doi.org/10.1080/10253890.2021.1891220.

256. Gukasyan and Narayan, "Menstrual Changes."

257. Derek Van Booven et al., "Alcohol Use Disorder Causes Global Changes in Splicing in the Human Brain," *Translational Psychiatry* 11, no. 1 (2021), https://doi.org/10.1038/s41398-020-01163-z.

258. Chong Min Goh et al., "Gender Differences in Alcohol Use: A Nationwide Study in a Multiethnic Population," *International Journal of Mental Health and Addiction* (2022), https://doi.org/10.1007/s11469-022-00921-y.

259. MacKenzie R. Peltier et al., "Sex Differences in Stress-Related Alcohol Use," *Neurobiology of Stress* 10 (2019), https://doi.org/10.1016/j.ynstr.2019.100149.

260. Peltier et al., "Sex Differences."

261. Goh et al., "Gender Differences in Alcohol Use."

262. Espen Lund Johannessen, Helle Wessel Andersson, Johan Håkon Bjørngaard, and Kristine Pape, "Anxiety and Depression Symptoms and Alcohol Use among Adolescents—A Cross Sectional Study of Norwegian Secondary School Students," *BMC Public Health* 17, no. 1 (2017), https://doi.org/10.1186/s12889-017-4389-2.

263. Peltier et al., "Sex Differences."

264. Peltier et al., "Sex Differences."

265. J. Gill, "The Effects of Moderate Alcohol Consumption on Female Hormone Levels and Reproductive Function," *Alcohol and Alcoholism* 35, no. 5 (2000): 417–23, https://doi.org/10.1093/alcalc/35.5.417.

266. Jill B. Becker and George F. Koob. "Sex Differences in Animal Models: Focus on Addiction," *Pharmacological Reviews* 68, no. 2 (2016): 242–63, https://doi.org/10.1124/pr.115.011163.

267. Michael P. Bogenschutz et al., "Percentage of Heavy Drinking Days Following Psilocybin-Assisted Psychotherapy vs Placebo in the Treatment of Adult Patients with Alcohol Use Disorder," *JAMA Psychiatry* 79, no. 10 (2022): 953, https://doi.org/10.1001/jamapsychiatry.2022.2096.

268. Bogenschutz et al., "Percentage of Heavy Drinking Days."

269. Bogenschutz et al., "Percentage of Heavy Drinking Days."

270. A. J. Baxter, K. M. Scott, T. Vos, and H. A. Whiteford, "Global Prevalence of Anxiety Disorders: A Systematic Review and Meta-Regression," *Psychological Medicine* 43, no. 5 (2012): 897–910, https://doi.org/10.1017/s003329171200147x.

271. Carmen P. McLean, Anu Asnaani, Brett T. Litz, and Stefan G. Hofmann, "Gender Differences in Anxiety Disorders: Prevalence, Course of Illness, Comorbidity and Burden of Illness," *Journal of Psychiatric Research* 45, no. 8 (2011): 1027–35. https://doi.org/10.1016/j.jpsychires.2011.03.006.

272. McLean et al., "Gender Differences in Anxiety Disorders."

273. McLean et al., "Gender Differences in Anxiety Disorders."

274. Maggie Kamila Kiraga et al., "Decreases in State and Trait Anxiety Post-Psilocybin: A Naturalistic, Observational Study among Retreat Attendees," *Frontiers in Psychiatry* 13 (2022), https://doi.org/10.3389/fpsyt.2022.883869.

275. Kiraga et al., "Decreases in State and Trait Anxiety."

276. Roland R. Griffiths et al., "Psilocybin Produces Substantial and Sustained Decreases in Depression and Anxiety in Patients with Life-Threatening Cancer: A Randomized Double-Blind Trial," *Journal of Psychopharmacology* 30, no. 12 (2016): 1181–97, https://doi.org/10.1177/0269881116675513.

277. Griffiths et al., "Psilocybin Produces Substantial."

278. Christopher R. Beam et al., "Differences between Women and Men in Incidence Rates of Dementia and Alzheimer's Disease," *Journal of Alzheimer's Disease* 64, no. 4 (2018): 1077–83, https://doi.org/10.3233/jad-180141.

279. Wenting Hao, Chunying Fu, and Dongshan Zhu, "Abstract EP67: Early Menopause Is Linked to Increased Risk of Presenile Dementia before Age 65 Years," *Circulation* 145 (2022), https://doi.org/10.1161/circ.145.suppl_1.ep67.

280. Albert Garcia-Romeu, and Paul B. Rosenberg. "Psilocybin for Depression in People with Mild Cognitive Impairment or Early Alzheimer's Disease," ClinicalTrials.gov, October 10, 2019, https://clinicaltrials.gov/ct2/show/NCT04123314.

281. Simon Andrew Vann Jones and Allison O'Kelly, "Psychedelics as a Treatment for Alzheimer's Disease Dementia," *Frontiers in Synaptic Neuroscience* 12 (2020), https://doi.org/10.3389/fnsyn.2020.00034.

282. Christine Kuehner, "Why Is Depression More Common among Women than among Men?" *The Lancet Psychiatry* 4, no. 2 (2017): 146–58, https://doi.org/10.1016/s2215-0366(16)30263-2.

283. Paul R. Albert, "Why Is Depression More Prevalent in Women?" *Journal of Psychiatry and Neuroscience* 40, no. 4 (2015): 219–21, https://doi.org/10.1503/jpn.150205.

284. Guy M. Goodwin et al., "Single-Dose Psilocybin for a Treatment-Resistant Episode of Major Depression," *New England Journal of Medicine* 387, no. 18 (2022): 1637–48, https://doi.org/10.1056/nejmoa2206443.

285. Goodwin et al., "Psilocybin for a Treatment-Resistant Episode."

286. Alan K. Davis et al., "Effects of Psilocybin-Assisted Therapy on Major Depressive Disorder," *JAMA Psychiatry* 78, no. 5 (2021): 481, https://doi.org/10.1001/jamapsychiatry.2020.3285.

287. Davis et al., "Effects of Psilocybin-Assisted Therapy."

288. Davis et al., "Effects of Psilocybin-Assisted Therapy."

289. Natalie Gukasyan et al., "Efficacy and Safety of Psilocybin-Assisted Treatment for Major Depressive Disorder: Prospective 12-Month Follow-Up," *Journal of Psychopharmacology* 36, no. 2 (2022): 151–58, https://doi.org/10.1177/02698811211073759.

290. "Information by Eating Disorder," National Eating Disorders Association, February 21, 2018, https://www.nationaleatingdisorders.org/information-eating -disorder.

291. Jie Qian et al., "An Update on the Prevalence of Eating Disorders in the General Population: A Systematic Review and Meta-Analysis," *Eating and Weight Disorders— Studies on Anorexia, Bulimia and Obesity* 27, no. 2 (2021): 415–28, https://doi.org/10 .1007/s40519-021-01162-z.

292. Meg J. Spriggs et al., "Study Protocol for 'Psilocybin as a Treatment for Anorexia Nervosa: A Pilot Study,'" *Frontiers in Psychiatry* 12 (2021), https://doi.org/10 .3389/fpsyt.2021.735523.

293. Imperial College London, "Psilocybin as a Treatment," ClinicalTrials.gov, NCT04505189.

294. "Psilocybin as a Treatment for Anorexia Nervosa: A Pilot Study," ClinicalTrials .gov, last updated October 3, 2022, https://clinicaltrials.gov/ct2/show/NCT04505189.

295. "Study Protocol for 'Psilocybin.'"

296. Andrea Phillipou, Susan L. Rossell, David J. Castle, and Caroline Gurvich, "Interoceptive Awareness in Anorexia Nervosa," *Journal of Psychiatric Research* 148 (2022): 84–87, https://doi.org/10.1016/j.jpsychires.2022.01.051.

297. Natalie Gukasyan, Colleen C. Schreyer, Roland R. Griffiths, and Angela S. Guarda, "Psychedelic-Assisted Therapy for People with Eating Disorders," *Current Psychiatry Reports* (2022), https://doi.org/10.1007/s11920-022-01394-5.

298. Phillipou et al., "Interoceptive Awareness."

299. Gukasyan et al., "Eating Disorders."

300. Gukasyan et al., "Eating Disorders."

301. Gukasyan et al., "Eating Disorders."

302. Ellis, Munro, and Clarke, "Endometriosis Is Undervalued."

303. Camran Nezhat et al., "Bilateral Thoracic Endometriosis Affecting the Lung and Diaphragm," *Journal of the Society of Laparoendoscopic Surgeons* 16, no. 1 (2012): 140–42, https://doi.org/10.4293/108680812x13291597716384.

304. Ellis, Munro, and Clarke, "Endometriosis Is Undervalued."

305. Silvia Vannuccini and Felice Petraglia, "Recent Advances in Understanding and Managing Adenomyosis," *F1000Research* 8 (2019): 283, https://doi.org/10.12688 /f1000research.17242.1.

306. Gukasyan and Narayan, "Menstrual Changes."

307. Clare Watson, "The Psychedelic Remedy for Chronic Pain," *Nature* 609, no. 7929 (2022), https://doi.org/10.1038/d41586-022-02878-3.

308. Sanah Malomile Nkadimeng, Christiaan M. L. Steinmann, and Jacobus N. Eloff, "Anti-Inflammatory Effects of Four Psilocybin-Containing Magic Mushroom Water Extracts in Vitro on 15-Lipoxygenase Activity and on Lipopolysaccharide-Induced Cyclooxygenase-2 and Inflammatory Cytokines in Human U937 Macrophage Cells," *Journal of Inflammation Research* 14 (2021): 3729–38, https://doi.org/10.2147/jir .s317182.

309. Nkadimeng, Steinmann, and Eloff, "Anti-Inflammatory Effects."

310. Mingyang Jiang et al., "The Efficacy and Safety of Selective COX-2 Inhibitors for Postoperative Pain Management in Patients after Total Knee/Hip Arthroplasty: A Meta-Analysis," *Journal of Orthopaedic Surgery and Research* 15, no. 1 (2020), https://doi.org/10.1186/s13018-020-1569-z.

311. Nkadimeng, Steinmann, and Eloff, "Anti-Inflammatory Effects."
312. Yi-Heng Lin et al., "Chronic Niche Inflammation in Endometriosis-Associated Infertility: Current Understanding and Future Therapeutic Strategies," *International Journal of Molecular Sciences* 19, no. 8 (2018): 2385. https://doi.org/10.3390/ijms19082385.
313. Lin et al., "Chronic Niche Inflammation in Endometriosis."
314. Massimo E. Maffei, "Fibromyalgia: Recent Advances in Diagnosis, Classification, Pharmacotherapy and Alternative Remedies," *International Journal of Molecular Sciences* 21, no. 21 (2020): 7877, https://doi.org/10.3390/ijms21217877.
315. Winfried Häuser and Mary-Ann Fitzcharles, "Facts and Myths Pertaining to Fibromyalgia," *Dialogues in Clinical Neuroscience* 20, no. 1 (2018): 53–62, https://doi.org/10.31887/dcns.2018.20.1/whauser.
316. Häuser and Fitzcharles, "Facts and Myths."
317. Peter Hendricks, "Psilocybin-Facilitated Treatment for Chronic Pain," ClinicalTrials.gov, last updated October 3, 2022. https://clinicaltrials.gov/ct2/show/NCT05068791.
318. Nicolas G. Glynos et al., "Knowledge, Perceptions, and Use of Psychedelics among Individuals with Fibromyalgia," *Journal of Psychoactive Drugs* (2022): 1–12, https://doi.org/10.1080/02791072.2021.2022817.
319. Glynos et al., "Knowledge, Perceptions, and Use."
320. Alisa Johnson, Lynae Roberts, and Gary Elkins, "Complementary and Alternative Medicine for Menopause," *Journal of Evidence-Based Integrative Medicine* 24 (2019), https://doi.org/10.1177/2515690x19829380.
321. Ellen B. Gold, "The Timing of the Age at Which Natural Menopause Occurs," *Obstetrics and Gynecology Clinics of North America* 38, no. 3 (2011): 425–40, https://doi.org/10.1016/j.ogc.2011.05.002.
322. Nanette Santoro, "Perimenopause: From Research to Practice," *Journal of Women's Health* 25, no. 4 (2016): 332–39, https://doi.org/10.1089/jwh.2015.5556.
323. Ellen W. Freeman, Mary D. Sammel, Hui Lin, and Clarisa R. Gracia, "Anti-Mullerian Hormone as a Predictor of Time to Menopause in Late Reproductive Age Women," *The Journal of Clinical Endocrinology & Metabolism* 97, no. 5 (2012): 1673–80, https://doi.org/10.1210/jc.2011-3032.
324. Santoro, "Perimenopause."
325. Santoro, "Perimenopause."
326. Henry Burger, "The Menopausal Transition—Endocrinology," *The Journal of Sexual Medicine* 5, no. 10 (2008): 2266–73, https://doi.org/10.1111/j.1743-6109.2008.00921.x.
327. "Depression & Menopause," Menopause.org, accessed December 7, 2022, https://www.menopause.org/for-women/menopauseflashes/mental-health-at-menopause/depression-menopause.
328. Lee S. Cohen et al., "Risk for New Onset of Depression during the Menopausal Transition," *Archives of General Psychiatry* 63, no. 4 (2006): 385, https://doi.org/10.1001/archpsyc.63.4.385.
329. Jessica A. Harder et al., "Brain-Derived Neurotrophic Factor and Mood in Perimenopausal Depression," *Journal of Affective Disorders* 300 (2022): 145–49, https://doi.org/10.1016/j.jad.2021.12.092.

330. Ekta Kapoor et al., "Association of Adverse Childhood Experiences with Menopausal Symptoms: Results from the Data Registry on Experiences of Aging, Menopause and Sexuality (Dreams)," *Maturitas* 143 (2021): 209–15, https://doi.org/10.1016/j.maturitas.2020.10.006.

331. Jennifer Chesak, "Can Trauma Affect Our Metabolic Health?" Levels Health, last updated September 30, 2022, https://www.levelshealth.com/blog/can-trauma-affect-our-metabolic-health.

332. Huseyin Cengiz, Cihan Kaya, Sema Suzen Caypinar, and Ismail Alay, "The Relationship between Menopausal Symptoms and Metabolic Syndrome in Postmenopausal Women," *Journal of Obstetrics and Gynaecology* 39, no. 4 (2019): 529–33, https://doi.org/10.1080/01443615.2018.1534812.

333. Monica De Paoli, Alexander Zakharia, and Geoff H. Werstuck, "The Role of Estrogen in Insulin Resistance," *The American Journal of Pathology* 191, no. 9 (2021): 1490–98, https://doi.org/10.1016/j.ajpath.2021.05.011.

334. Substance Abuse and Mental Health Services Administration, "People at Greater Risk of Suicide," SAMHSA.gov, accessed November 12, 2022, https://www.samhsa.gov/suicide/at-risk.

335. Jayashri Kulkarni, "Perimenopausal Depression—An Under-Recognised Entity," *Australian Prescriber* 41, no. 6 (2018): 183–85, https://doi.org/10.18773/austprescr.2018.060.

336. "Does Depression Increase the Risk for Suicide?" HHS.gov, October 20, 2021, https://www.hhs.gov/answers/mental-health-and-substance-abuse/does-depression-increase-risk-of-suicide/index.html.

337. Goodwin et al., "Psilocybin for a Treatment-Resistant Episode."

338. Linda Al-Hassany et al., "Giving Researchers a Headache—Sex and Gender Differences in Migraine," *Frontiers in Neurology* 11 (2020), https://doi.org/10.3389/fneur.2020.549038.

339. American Migraine Foundation, "Menstrual Migraine Treatment and Prevention," American Migraine Foundation, October 3, 2022, https://americanmigrainefoundation.org/resource-library/menstrual-migraine-treatment-and-prevention.

340. Emmanuelle A. Schindler et al., "Exploratory Controlled Study of the Migraine-Suppressing Effects of Psilocybin," *Neurotherapeutics* 18, no. 1 (2020): 534–43, https://doi.org/10.1007/s13311-020-00962-y.

341. Schindler et al., "Migraine-Suppressing Effects of Psilocybin."

342. Watson, "Psychedelic Remedy for Chronic Pain."

343. Carla Dugas and Valori H Slane. "Miscarriage," In *StatsPearls*, Treasure Island, FL: StatPearls Publishing, 2022, https://www.ncbi.nlm.nih.gov/books/NBK532992.

344. Siobhan Quenby et al., "Miscarriage Matters: The Epidemiological, Physical, Psychological, and Economic Costs of Early Pregnancy Loss," *The Lancet* 397, no. 10285 (2021): 1658–67, https://doi.org/10.1016/s0140-6736(21)00682-6.

345. Quenby et al., "Miscarriage Matters."

346. Bruno Aouizerate et al., "Pathophysiology of Obsessive–Compulsive Disorder," *Progress in Neurobiology* 72, no. 3 (2004): 195–221, https://doi.org/10.1016/j.pneurobio.2004.02.004.

347. Emily J. Fawcett, Hilary Power, and Jonathan M. Fawcett, "Women Are at Greater Risk of OCD than Men," *The Journal of Clinical Psychiatry* 81, no. 4 (2020), https://doi.org/10.4088/jcp.19r13085.

348. Griffiths, "Psilocybin in Obsessive Compulsive Disorder," ClinicalTrials.gov, NCT05546658; Benjamin Kelmendi, "Efficacy of Psilocybin in OCD: A Double-Blind, Placebo-Controlled Study," ClinicalTrials.gov, last updated December 9, 2021, https://clinicaltrials.gov/ct2/show/NCT03356483.

349. Francisco A. Moreno, Christopher B. Wiegand, E. Keolani Taitano, and Pedro L. Delgado, "Safety, Tolerability, and Efficacy of Psilocybin in 9 Patients with Obsessive-Compulsive Disorder," *The Journal of Clinical Psychiatry* 67, no. 11 (2006): 1735–40, https://doi.org/10.4088/jcp.v67n1110.

350. Moreno et al., "Safety, Tolerability, and Efficacy of Psilocybin in 9 Patients."

351. Alexander M. Dydyk, Mohit Gupta, and Nitesh K. Jain, "Opioid Use Disorder," in StatsPearls, Treasure Island, FL: StatPearls Publishing, 2022, https://www.ncbi.nlm.nih.gov/books/NBK553166.

352. Mikkael Sekeres, "When Patients Need Opioids to Ease the Pain," *New York Times*, July 10, 2019, https://www.nytimes.com/2019/07/10/well/live/when-patients-need-opioids-to-ease-the-pain.html.

353. Yvon Yeo, Rosemary Johnson, and Christine Heng, "The Public Health Approach to the Worsening Opioid Crisis in the United States Calls for Harm Reduction Strategies to Mitigate the Harm from Opioid Addiction and Overdose Deaths," *Military Medicine* 187, no. 9-10 (2021): 244–47, https://doi.org/10.1093/milmed/usab485.

354. Karin Mack, Linda Frazier, and Mishka Trepan, "Addressing the Unique Challenges of Opioid Use Disorder in Women," Centers for Disease Control and Prevention, January 17, 2017, https://www.cdc.gov/grand-rounds/pp/2017/20170117-opioid-overdose.html.

355. Teddy G. Goetz, Jill B. Becker, and Carolyn M. Mazure, "Women, Opioid Use and Addiction," *The FASEB Journal* 35, no. 2 (2021), https://doi.org/10.1096/fj.202002125r.

356. Serdarevic, Striley, and Cottler, "Sex Differences in Prescription Opioid."

357. Vincent D. Pisano et al., "The Association of Psychedelic Use and Opioid Use Disorders among Illicit Users in the United States," *Journal of Psychopharmacology* 31, no. 5 (2017): 606–13, https://doi.org/10.1177/0269881117691453.

358. Albert Garcia-Romeu et al., "Persisting Reductions in Cannabis, Opioid, and Stimulant Misuse after Naturalistic Psychedelic Use: An Online Survey," *Frontiers in Psychiatry* 10 (2020), https://doi.org/10.3389/fpsyt.2019.00955.

359. Jones et al., "Classic Psychedelics and Opioid Use Disorder."

360. Jones et al., "Classic Psychedelics and Opioid Use Disorder."

361. Matthew W. Johnson, "Psilocybin for Opioid Use Disorder in Patients on Methadone Maintenance with Ongoing Opioid Use," ClinicalTrials.gov, last updated October 24, 2022, https://clinicaltrials.gov/ct2/show/NCT05242029.

362. Saba Mughal, Yusra Azhar, and Waquar Siddiqui, "Postpartum Depression," in *StatPearls*. Treasure Island, FL: StatPearls, 2022, https://www.ncbi.nlm.nih.gov/books/NBK519070.

363. Elizabeth Q. Cox, Nathaniel A. Sowa, Samantha E. Meltzer-Brody, and Bradley N. Gaynes, "The Perinatal Depression Treatment Cascade," *The Journal of Clinical Psychiatry* 77, no. 9 (2016): 1189–1200, https://doi.org/10.4088/jcp.15r10174.

364. Payne and Maguire, "Mechanisms Implicated in Postpartum Depression."

365. Chaitra Jairaj, and James J Rucker, "Postpartum Depression: A Role for Psychedelics?" *Journal of Psychopharmacology* 36, no. 8 (2022): 920–31, https://doi.org/10.1177/02698811221093793.

366. Slomian et al., "Consequences of Maternal Postpartum Depression."

367. Jennifer L. Payne and Jamie Maguire. "Pathophysiological Mechanisms Implicated in Postpartum Depression," *Frontiers in Neuroendocrinology* 52 (2019): 165–80, https://doi.org/10.1016/j.yfrne.2018.12.001.

368. Jairaj and Rucker, "Postpartum Depression."

369. Jairaj and Rucker, "Postpartum Depression."

370. Melissa Lavasani and Beth Dreher, "Magic Mushrooms Helped Me Cope with My Severe Postpartum Depression," *Good Housekeeping*, June 10, 2021, https://www.goodhousekeeping.com/health/wellness/a35681767/magic-mushrooms-postpartum-depression.

371. Maria Brus Pedersen, "I Ate Psychedelic Mushrooms to Treat My Postpartum Depression," *VICE*, January 25, 2019, https://www.vice.com/en/article/zmdvjy/microdosing-magic-mushrooms-postpartum-depression-treatment.

372. Julie Ugleholdt *Projekt Baby: Mit Første År Som Uperfekt Mor*, Pink Moon, 2018.

373. National Institute of Mental Health, "Post-Traumatic Stress Disorder."

374. Elsouri et al., "Psychoactive Drugs."

375. Olff, "Sex and Gender Differences."

376. Bradley D. Grinage, "Diagnosis and Management of Post-Traumatic Stress Disorder," *American Family Physician* 68, no. 12 (2003): 2401–8.

377. Olff, "Sex and Gender Differences."

378. Gosia, "Investigating the Therapeutic Effects."

379. Elsouri et al., "Psychoactive Drugs."

380. Elsouri et al., "Psychoactive Drugs."

381. Sanskriti Mishra, Harold Elliott, and Raman Marwaha," Premenstrual Dysphoric Disorder—Statpearls—NCBI Bookshelf," in *StatPearls*. Treasure Island, FL: StatPearl, 2022, https://www.ncbi.nlm.nih.gov/books/NBK532307.

382. Teresa Lanza di Scalea and Teri Pearlstein, "Premenstrual Dysphoric Disorder," *Psychiatric Clinics of North America* 40, no. 2 (2017): 201–16, https://doi.org/10.1016/j.psc.2017.01.002.

383. Peter J. Schmidt et al., "Premenstrual Dysphoric Disorder Symptoms Following Ovarian Suppression: Triggered by Change in Ovarian Steroid Levels but Not Continuous Stable Levels," *American Journal of Psychiatry* 174, no. 10 (2017): 980–89, https://doi.org/10.1176/appi.ajp.2017.16101113.

384. Liisa Hantsoo and C. Neill Epperson, "Premenstrual Dysphoric Disorder: Epidemiology and Treatment," *Current Psychiatry Reports* 17, no. 11 (2015), https://doi.org/10.1007/s11920-015-0628-3.

385. Sara V. Carlini and Kristina M. Deligiannidis, "Evidence-Based Treatment of Premenstrual Dysphoric Disorder," *The Journal of Clinical Psychiatry* 81, no. 2 (2020), https://doi.org/10.4088/jcp.19ac13071.

386. Stephen M. Stahl, "Mechanism of Action of Serotonin Selective Reuptake Inhibitors," *Journal of Affective Disorders* 51, no. 3 (1998): 215–35, https://doi.org/10.1016/s0165-0327(98)00221-3.

387. Hantsoo and Epperson, "Premenstrual Dysphoric Disorder."

388. Castelhano et al., "Effects of Tryptamine Psychedelics."

389. Gukasyan and Narayan, "Menstrual Changes."

390. Carissa R. Violante, "Draw an Informed Conclusion: Why Is It Harder for Women to Quit Smoking?" Yale School of Medicine, November 14, 2016, https://medicine.yale

.edu/news-article/draw-an-informed-conclusion-why-is-it-harder-for-women-to-quit
-smoking.

391. Ami P. Raval, "Nicotine Addiction Causes Unique Detrimental Effects on Women's Brains," *Journal of Addictive Diseases* 30, no. 2 (2011): 149–58, https://doi .org/10.1080/10550887.2011.554782.

392. Tony Hicks, "Nicotine Blocks Estrogen in Women's Brains, Making It Harder to Quit Smoking," *Healthline*, October 17, 2022, https://www.healthline.com/health-news /nicotine-may-block-estrogen-in-womens-brains-making-it-harder-to-quit-smoking #Studying-the-synthesis-of-estrogen-in-the-brain.Z

393. Jonas Crabtree, "How Quitting Smoking Is Different for Women," SEARHC.org, January 13, 2020, https://searhc.org/how-quitting-smoking-is-different-for-women.

394. Matthew W. Johnson, Albert Garcia-Romeu, Mary P. Cosimano, and Roland R. Griffiths, "Pilot Study of the 5-HT2aR Agonist Psilocybin in the Treatment of Tobacco Addiction," *Journal of Psychopharmacology* 28, no. 11 (2014): 983–92, https://doi.org /10.1177/0269881114548296.

395. Matthew W. Johnson and Roland R. Griffiths, "Potential Therapeutic Effects of Psilocybin," *Neurotherapeutics* 14, no. 3 (2017): 734–40, https://doi.org/10.1007 /s13311-017-0542-y.

396. Tehseen Noorani et al., "Psychedelic Therapy for Smoking Cessation: Qualitative Analysis of Participant Accounts," *Journal of Psychopharmacology* 32, no. 7 (2018): 756–69, https://doi.org/10.1177/0269881118780612.

397. Osiris Sinuhé González Romero, "María Sabina, Mushrooms, and Colonial Extractivism," Chacruna.net, May 27, 2021, https://chacruna.net/maria-sabina -mushrooms-and-colonial-extractivism.

398. Robert Gordon Wasson, "1957 - Wasson—Life Magazine—Secret of Divine Mushrooms (Web) PDF," *Life*, May 13, 1957, https://www.scribd.com/document /476539657/1957-Wasson-Life-Magazine-Secret-of-Divine-Mushrooms-web-pdf.

399. "Some Historical Figures Who Visited Oaxacan María Sabina, the Great Mexican Shaman," *The Oaxaca Post*, February 7, 2022, https://theoaxacapost.com/2022/02 /07/some-historical-figures-who-visited-oaxacan-maria-sabina-the-great-mexican -shaman.

400. "Psymposia," accessed December 7, 2022, https://www.psymposia.com.

ACKNOWLEDGMENTS

I owe a debt of gratitude to the friends and family who've championed me along this writing journey and who always nourish me with love, support, and comic relief. You know who you are. I'm a lucky gal to have you in my corner. Please know I'm always in yours.

Thanks to Gabriel Castillo and Bridgette Rivera of Finally Detached for holding space for me and crafting such a beautiful retreat where I could truly lean in to my first psilocybin experience. It was magical!

This book would not be possible without the generosity of time and expertise from the people who agreed to be interviewed for these pages. I'm grateful to all of you.

Many thanks to the entire team at Ulysses Press, especially associate editor Kierra Sondereker who took me on for this exciting project, senior managing editor Renee Rutledge who shuttled me through the many steps of the final stretch, and Scott Calamar who copyedited the manuscript.

Thank you to all the editors over the years who've given my words a home at various publications and who've helped me grow as a journalist. I appreciate you and your work!

Special thanks to Michael Mann for always being a sounding board for writing, editing, and life conundrums.

Sara, thank you for "breaking me out" of the hospital that one time. I'll never forget that, and this is a thank-you for so much more, including sharing your family with me.

Gratitude to my husband, Jereme, for keeping me entertained, in good coffee and edibles, health-insured, and on a reasonable schedule—all things this night owl and freelancer needs. Thank you for being you and never interfering with me being me. Also, thanks for the amazing in-laws and Josh Posh and Co.

A huge thanks to my mom and dad for always championing my journalistic endeavors. (Yes, even when I told you I was writing a book about drugs!) As we say in our family, I love you muches.

Finally, a special thanks to the late Fiver, aka Juni, who was always a balm to any pain. Your memory will always be.

ABOUT the AUTHOR

Jennifer Chesak is an award-winning freelance science and medical journalist, editor, and fact-checker based in Nashville, Tennessee. Her work has appeared in the *Washington Post*, Healthline, Verywell Health, Health, Better Homes and Gardens, Greatist, Parents, mindbodygreen, Levels, *B*tch*, Sleep.com, and more. Her coverage focuses on chronic health issues, medical rights, health care, harm reduction, and the scientific evidence around health and wellness trends, including cannabis and psychedelics.

Jennifer earned her master of science in journalism from Northwestern University's Medill. She currently teaches in the journalism and publishing programs at Belmont University, leads various workshops at the literary nonprofit The Porch, and serves as the managing editor for the literary magazine *SHIFT*. In her free time, Jennifer, who is originally from North Dakota, can be found covered in mud out on a trail run or in her garden. Find her work at jenniferchesak.com and follow her on socials @jenchesak.

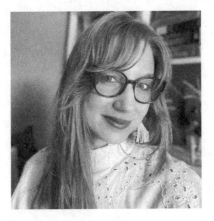